Publishing and Presenting
Clinical Research

THIRD EDITION

WARREN S. BROWNER, MD, MPH
Chief Executive Officer
California Pacific Medical Center
Adjunct Professor of Epidemiology & Biostatistics
University of California, San Francisco
San Francisco, California

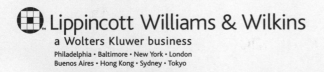
. Lippincott Williams & Wilkins
a Wolters Kluwer business
Philadelphia · Baltimore · New York · London
Buenos Aires · Hong Kong · Sydney · Tokyo

Senior Acquisitions Editor: Sonya Seigafuse
Senior Product Manager: Kerry Barrett
Vendor Manager: Bridgett Dougherty
Senior Manufacturing Manager: Benjamin Rivera
Senior Marketing Manager: Kim Schonberger
Design Coordinator: Joan Wendt
Production Service: S4Carlisle Publishing Services

© 2012 by LIPPINCOTT WILLIAMS & WILKINS, a WOLTERS KLUWER business
Two Commerce Square
2001 Market Street
Philadelphia, PA 19103 USA
LWW.com

Printed in China

Library of Congress Cataloging-in-Publication Data

Browner, Warren S.
Publishing and presenting clinical research / Warren S. Browner.—3rd ed.
    p. ; cm.
Includes bibliographical references and index.
ISBN-13: 978-1-4511-1590-1
ISBN-10: 1-4511-1590-3
I. Title.
[DNLM: 1. Publishing. 2. Biomedical Research. 3. Periodicals as Topic. 4. Writing. WZ 345]
LC classification not assigned
808'.06661—dc23

2011049231

Care has been taken to confirm the accuracy of the information presented and to describe generally accepted practices. However, the authors, editors, and publisher are not responsible for errors or omissions or for any consequences from application of the information in this book and make no warranty, expressed or implied, with respect to the currency, completeness, or accuracy of the contents of the publication. Application of the information in a particular situation remains the professional responsibility of the practitioner.

To purchase additional copies of this book, call our customer service department at (800) 638-3030 or fax orders to (301) 223-2320. International customers should call (301) 223-2300.

Visit Lippincott Williams & Wilkins on the Internet: at LWW.com. Lippincott Williams & Wilkins customer service representatives are available from 8:30 am to 6 pm, EST.

10 9 8 7 6 5 4 3 2 1

To my family, friends, and colleagues, with gratitude

Contents

Acknowledgments

I was lucky enough to have Steve Hulley and Steve Cummings as mentors early in my research career, which is a little bit like waking up on third base and thinking you've hit a triple. Years later, I had the opportunity to work with several wonderful colleagues, including Lee Goldman, editing the American Journal of Medicine. All of them understood that how you present something matters almost as much as what you present. This book is an attempt to provide a practical approach for investigators who struggle with putting their thoughts into words and pictures, and who do not have someone nearby who can help.

Overview

WHO SHOULD USE THIS BOOK?

If you are like most investigators, you may have difficulty making the transition from consumers to producers of medical literature. Perhaps you are intimidated at the prospect of committing your ideas and the results of your research into a formal written document—how can your work possibly be up to the standards of the scientific community? After all, most new clinical investigators were first introduced to the medical literature at journal clubs, in which you and your colleagues searched exhaustively to find all the problems in the articles that were discussed. As a result, you may feel compelled to produce a perfect manuscript or you may have a ton of data but not a clue about how to begin. It may also be that you are in the unfortunate spot of having a manuscript or two that you just cannot finish, or need to make a presentation at an upcoming meeting. In any event, if you have read this far, it is likely that you have found yourself needing some help. Welcome to a large group of other investigators. I hope you find what you are looking for in the next 200 pages or so.

In addition to helping you get started (and finished!) with your manuscripts and presentations, this book will give you guidance on getting your work accepted in medical journals and at scientific meetings. Sometimes relatively small changes in what you write, or how you have written it, can make the difference between a manuscript that leads to a response that says, "Sorry, we receive thousands of submissions each year and thus must turn away most of them" and one that gets accepted at the journal of your choice.

Perhaps you have more abstracts than publications in your curriculum vitae, or you cannot "break through" to the better journals in your field because you struggle as a writer. Perhaps your articles are rejected for stylistic reasons or because you have not been able to emphasize what is new and important about your study. Maybe you have had the experience of having everyone but the reviewers and journal editors tell you how important your work seems. Perhaps reviewers comment that your paper is "poorly written," "disorganized," or "lacks focus," and suggest that you find an editor.

Many authors find themselves wondering what to do about "negative" (nonsignificant) results. Chapter 5 provides some guidance about what to do in this situation.

Students, residents, and fellows working on research projects, and junior faculty who have received little or no formal training in presenting and publishing research, may also find this book useful. Many investigators are "undertrained" in clinical research, and do not really understand some of the basic concepts, such as effect size and confidence intervals or dealing with issues about authorship. If there are holes in your knowledge about the nuts and bolts of research, you will find much useful information in this book. Of course, a book about how to present your research—either orally or in writing—cannot possibly be a complete guide to design and execute a good research project. For that, I would encourage you to read a companion volume to this book, *Designing Clinical Research: An Epidemiologic Approach*,[1] by several colleagues in San Francisco.

This book will also help investigators for whom English is a second or third language. No matter how fluent you are, problems with English that cause no difficulty in informal verbal communication—because people can understand what you meant to say or can ask for clarification—can become grating errors in print or during a formal presentation. Non–English-speaking scientists face an additional difficulty. Reading articles in English is hard enough; discerning their underlying form and structure is nearly impossible. Non–English-speaking authors may therefore be less familiar with how a manuscript should look.

Perhaps you find yourself in the awkward position of being responsible for a manuscript or presentation that has more authors than collaborators. In other words, you need to figure out how to tell someone who wants to be an author on your manuscript (presumably because the results are worthwhile) that he or she does not qualify for that privilege. Read Chapter 10, and perhaps add a xeroxed copy of the penultimate paragraph in your mentor's mailbox.

Finally, this book is aimed at senior investigators who think they are spending too much time helping junior colleagues with manuscripts. Part of my motivation—as mentor, reviewer, and journal editor—has been trying to prevent the same mistakes from being repeated.

WHEN WILL THIS BOOK BE USEFUL?

You can use this book as you are getting ready to submit an abstract or present your results at a meeting. There are chapters on how to write an abstract (and how to shorten one), how to make posters and slides, and how to prepare a talk. If you have already begun to write a manuscript, then the book provides advice about how to write each section—from introduction to discussion. If your initial reaction to writing a manuscript resembles the effects of botulinum toxin on the neuromuscular system, you may find this step-by-step approach helpful.

Perhaps your manuscript is already written. You are readying it for submission to a journal and looking for a last-minute tune-up to enhance its acceptability. Could the tables and figures use some remodeling? Can the writing style be improved? What should the cover letter say? How should a response to the reviewers be prepared?

Finally, although this book does not provide specific guidance on assembling a grant proposal, many aspects of writing a manuscript and preparing a proposal are similar. The same principles that lead to a concise, focused manuscript will also improve a grant proposal. Given that most reviewers have to read a lot of grant proposals in a very short time, a proposal that is well written will more likely be rated highly. Conversely, a grant application that rambles aimlessly or fails to convey a clear message will almost certainly fail to be approved for funding.

HOW TO USE THIS BOOK

You can read the book cover to cover on your own, whether or not a manuscript or presentation looms. It may help to read it with a group of colleagues who review each other's abstracts as they are submitted, look at posters and presentations as they are prepared, and critique sections of manuscripts as they are written.

You might prefer to read one chapter at a time, as the need arises. When you are faced with an abstract that will not fit into its allocated space, or an introduction that refuses to write itself, or a table that just looks clumsy, you can draw on the examples in the book for some fresh ideas.

Finally, no matter how hard the task of preparing a manuscript seems, remember the most important rule: *Present your results*. As a clinical investigator, you have made a moral commitment. Subjects agreed to participate in your project with the expectation that they were contributing to science. Some of these people, such as those with a serious illness, may have participated in your research with the thought that it was their final chance to make a contribution to the betterment of humanity. Nearly all subjects in a medical research study take their participation very seriously. That means you have an obligation to publish your results or at least make a serious effort. This book provides some of the tools you will need to make that attempt your best possible effort.

Reference

1. Hulley SB, Cummings SR, Browner WS, et al., eds. *Designing Clinical Research: An Epidemiologic Approach*. 3rd ed. Philadelphia, PA: Lippincott Williams & Wilkins; 2007.

2   Title and Abstract

It may seem obvious to say so: Both the title and the abstract of your manuscript should focus on your research question. Why emphasize the importance of the research question in a book about writing, especially considering that the research question should have been set at the time the study was designed? Because many investigators, particularly at the beginning of their careers, are handed a pile of charts and analyses by a more senior colleague, with the vague instruction to "write this up." Make sure you are clear about the research question before you start that process.

What is a research question? Simply put, it is what you might say—between floors in an elevator—to a colleague who asks, "What are you studying?" A research question should be sufficiently sophisticated so that if the chair of your department happens to be riding on the same elevator, he will be impressed by your savvy. If your uncle should step aboard, he should also be able to understand your answer. The research question does not have to be in the form of a question—this is not *Jeopardy!* Here are a few examples of how you might answer your fellow passengers in the elevator:

> I'm studying whether a 3-day course of antibiotics is as effective as a 7-day course in treating impetigo in children.

> My study looks at whether patients with rheumatoid arthritis who have used non-steroidal anti-inflammatory agents are less likely to develop rheumatoid lung disease.

> My research question focuses on determining whether a new blood test can identify which patients with chronic heart failure are at high risk for ventricular arrhythmias.

Once you have determined the research question, you need to identify the main features of your study that you want readers to remember. If you have more than five or six key points, it is going to be difficult—maybe even too difficult—to focus the paper. The features might include the type of study (e.g., a prospective cohort study), the subjects (e.g., elderly patients with hypertension), the main measurements (e.g., 72-hour ambulatory blood pressure monitoring), your analytic methods (e.g., adjustment for confounders using multivariable models) as well as the main result (e.g., that use of a beta blocker reduces lability of blood pressure). Many of these points should be noted in the title, and all of them must be covered in the abstract. Then, by reappearing throughout the manuscript, these points will give focus to your work.

THE TITLE

A title should be based on the research question. Beyond that, the more interesting the title, the better. The title should trigger a synapse in the minds of reviewers and readers who say, "Hey, that sounds interesting. I should read this." Conversely, your title must not lead to any of the following reactions: "Not again," "Cannot be," "How dull," or "Huh?"

A catchy title, if you can think of one, may encourage readers to at least dip into the paper ("Effects of stage migration on lung cancer mortality: The Will Rogers phenomenon"). However, avoid pretentiousness or dubious taste ("Evaluation of intracavernous phentolamine: The Mae West phenomenon"). When in doubt, choose a declarative title, such as "The association between A and B in C" or "The effect of A on B: Importance of C."

Try out several versions of the title on colleagues and coauthors. Ask coinvestigators who are knowledgeable about the study whether the title is accurate. Then ask persons who are not familiar with your study how much they can tell about it just from reading the title. Remember that the key features of your study (e.g., a clinical trial, children with ear infections, or a new antibiotic) should appear in the title. Certain words, including *novel, randomized, controlled, blinded,* and *prospective,* convey a certain panache if they appear—deservedly, of course—in a title.

Should the Title Be Bold?

Why not use an assertive title, such as "The ACE deletion genotype reduces survival after myocardial infarction," to draw the readers' attention. There are a few reasons, none of them absolute. First, bragging about your results may increase a reviewer's skepticism, especially if your findings contradict that reviewer's opinion. By contrast, a dispassionate-sounding title gives an aura of objectivity to the work. Another good reason to tone down your title applies to abstracts submitted to meetings, especially if the project is not entirely finished when you send in the abstract. Many investigators have seen their results change between the time an abstract was submitted and the time the results are presented at the meeting. It is somewhat less embarrassing if the title did not promise something that could not be delivered, even if the body of the abstract is wrong. Mostly, however, the decision about the objectivity of a title is a matter of style. If it is commonplace in your field to use flashy titles, then do so. If you are not sure, check recent journals or proceedings and phrase the title accordingly.

What Should I Do If My Study Is Not Very Original?

What should you do if your study is the fifth or tenth on the same topic? Should you title it, for example, "Yet another study of the association between hypertension and stroke"? Or perhaps "Measurement of arterial blood pressure using a sphygmomanometer as a way to identify patients at high risk for stroke"? Although choosing either of these titles might be a brave (albeit potentially career-limiting) decision, there are less drastic alternatives. Is there anything novel about your study? Perhaps your study marked the first time the association was studied in patients recovering from alcoholism. Is there anything particularly rigorous about the design of your study? Yours may have been the first study to use a new ambulatory blood pressure monitoring device. Is there anything surprising about your results? Perhaps you found that hypertension was not a risk factor for stroke in persons younger than 50 years. Special features of the study, if any, should be highlighted in the title.

Do Not Be Misleading

Readers of a study's title, whether they are flipping through the table of contents of a journal, glancing at the program for a scientific meeting, or doing a computerized literature search, will want to know to which species the study applies. If the identity of the study population is not clear, especially if it is not certain whether the subjects were humans or rodents, then it should be clarified. Human subjects are assumed unless stated otherwise. If you are studying rats, then say so in the title. In the same vein, if you studied a unique population (nursing home residents, Korean War veterans, or inner-city emergency room users), it should be mentioned in the title. The same goes for novel measurement methods, which should be noted if they were an important reason for the study.

What If I Cannot Think of a Title?

If you are still not sure what the title of your abstract or manuscript should be, fill in the following blank:

My study showed that_____.

Then generalize and reorder the phrase you used to fill in the blank. For example:

1. My study showed that women were more likely than men to discuss diet and exercise with their doctors becomes the following title:

    Effects of Patient Sex on Communication about Lifestyle with Physicians

2. My study showed that after adjusting for age, women were not more likely than men to discuss diet and exercise with their doctors becomes:

    Effects of Patient Sex on Communication with Physicians Are Confounded by Age.

3. My study showed that treatment with mouthwash reduced the incidence of thrush becomes:

    A Randomized Blinded Trial of Mouthwash in the Prevention of Oral Candidiasis

4. My study showed that patients with the ACE deletion genotype were less likely to survive after a myocardial infarction becomes:

    Association between ACE Deletion Genotype and Survival after Myocardial Infarction

 ## ABSTRACTS

Abstracts come in two main types: those submitted to scientific meetings and those that accompany full-length articles. Each type has different functions.

An abstract submitted to a meeting will be reviewed for scientific quality, relevance, and interest. The only information that reviewers will have about your study—and its results—will be what you can fit into the abstract. Make sure to include an overview of the study as well as any critical methodologic details, as discussed in the next several pages.

Abstracts submitted with a manuscript have a less essential function because reviewers and readers have the rest of the paper to fill in any gaps. They simply serve as a summary of the manuscript. A poorly written abstract will not eliminate an entire manuscript from consideration, whereas a poor abstract submitted to a meeting is doomed. However, once a manuscript is published, the abstract often serves as the paper's "representative" on the Internet (and for readers who do not have access to the full paper, it is the only information they will have about your study), so it is worth ensuring that the abstract is written well.

PREPARING AN ABSTRACT FOR A SCIENTIFIC MEETING

For most investigators, submitting an abstract to a scientific meeting is the first opportunity to have their work evaluated by peers. Early in your career, especially at the critical stage when you may be looking for your first faculty position, preparing an abstract serves several other important functions. It forces you to set aside data gathering for a while and synthesize your results. Often, that turns out to be a useful process, even if the abstract is not accepted. Writing an abstract can clarify the direction of your research. You may realize that essential parts of the study are incomplete or that more subjects are needed; or you may discover that the reason you are having such a difficult time summarizing your work in a single abstract is that you are actually doing two or more distinct projects. Best of all, if your abstract is accepted, you will have the opportunity to meet other investigators in your field (see Chapters 11 and 12 on posters and oral presentations on how to get the most out of presenting your results). But do not delay writing the full manuscript while waiting to hear whether an abstract has been accepted.

Most of all, submitting an abstract to a meeting will also provide you with a valuable clue as to the merit of your work. Although many investigators have a story about a rejected abstract or a 5:30 PM poster presentation that was later published in a prestigious journal, do not count on that happening to you. The response to your full-length manuscript when you submit it for publication will usually parallel the response to the abstract that you submitted to a meeting. The best abstracts at a scientific meeting are chosen for so-called plenary sessions, which are scheduled for the main auditorium at times when there are no other competing events. Abstracts rated next highest are selected for oral presentations, which are talks with slides lasting 10 or 15 minutes. Next in order of prestige are poster presentations, in which you prepare a poster describing your work, attach it to a bulletin board, and stand by it for a few hours during the meeting, discussing your research with passersby. Least prestigious are abstracts that were not accepted; these may, however, be published in the proceedings of the meeting.

How Do I List Abstracts in My Curriculum Vitae?

This pecking order has given rise to the practice of trying to indicate on your curriculum vitae (CV) how well your abstract did. The shorter your CV, the more important these distinctions are.

Hart A, Quandt Z. The definitive study of the relative worth of abstracts at scientific meetings. Presented in plenary session at *Sixth International Meeting of the Society of Medical Publishing.* Galveston; 2010; *J Int Soc Med Publ.* 2010;12(S):67. (The clues that this presentation was a big deal are the words international and plenary.)

White S, Fisher J. A very good study of the relative worth of abstracts at scientific meetings. *Oral Presentation at Fourth National Meeting of the Society of Medical Publishing.* Poughkeepsie; 2010; *J Am Soc Med Publ.* 2010;12(S):75. (Here, the clues are oral and national.)

Hunter A, Crane A. An adequate study of the relative worth of abstracts at scientific meetings. Presented at *Second Northwestern Regional Meeting of the Society of Medical Publishing.* Portland; 2010; *J Am Soc Med Publ.* 2010;12(S):118. (This was probably a poster presentation.)

Watkins H, Halperin RJ. A not-so-hot study of the relative worth of abstracts at scientific meetings. *J Am Soc Med Publ.* 2010;12(S):244. (This may not even have been presented as a poster).

It is unlikely that this last group of authors will convince a major journal to accept the manuscript describing their work. The authors who made a plenary presentation stand a much better chance.

How Do I Decide Whether to Submit One Abstract or Two?

Commonly, new investigators are uncertain whether they have "enough stuff" to warrant submitting an abstract. A related concern is whether they have too much information for a single abstract; perhaps two would be better. There are no established guidelines for making these determinations; common sense and talking with mentors can provide some guidance. The best rule is "One abstract per research question, and one research question per abstract." In most circumstances, it is also true that each abstract should be able to support a unique manuscript. If two abstracts have similar background and methods sections, they probably should be combined into a single abstract that discusses a few predictor variables associated with a given outcome or a few outcome variables associated with a given predictor. (If you do not know what predictor and outcome variables are, see *Designing Clinical Research: An Epidemiologic Approach.*[1] In the first example below, diabetes and hypercholesterolemia are predictors; morbidity and mortality following surgery are outcomes.) For example,

Change:

1. Diabetes increases morbidity following carotid endarterectomy and

2. Mortality after carotid artery surgery is related to preoperative cholesterol level.

To:

Effects of diabetes and hypercholesterolemia on outcome after carotid surgery.

Change:

1. Level of education and the incidence of stroke in Hispanic Americans, and

2. Educational levels in Hispanic Americans and the risk of coronary heart disease.

To:

Level of education and cardiovascular outcomes in Hispanic Americans.

However, if you are having a difficult time organizing your abstract or deciding on a title, it is often a clue that your subject may be too broad and should be divided into two or more abstracts. An abstract that tries to cover too much, or disparate topics, should be split in two.

Change:

Psychological and hematologic predictors of survival with leukemia

To:

1. Psychological factors associated with poor prognosis in leukemia, and

2. Survival with leukemia: Hematologic markers.

What If Colleagues Want to Submit Abstracts on the Same Topic?

Another problem may arise when several investigators want to submit abstracts from the same study, each taking a turn as first author, second author, and so on. This strategy has the apparent advantage of providing each of the authors with several other abstracts for their CVs. A senior author, who serves as the final author for the entire group, may even encourage this lamentable practice:

McDonald K, Baron H, Adler S, Bigshot Q. Ventilation–perfusion mismatches in patients with idiopathic pulmonary fibrosis. Presented at the *Annual Meeting of the American Society of Pulmonologists...*

Baron H, Adler S, McDonald K, Bigshot Q. Idiopathic pulmonary fibrosis: Evidence that ventilation and perfusion may be mismatched. Presented at the *International Meeting of the Nuclear Medicine Association...*

Adler S, McDonald K, Baron H, Bigshot Q. Are problems in ventilation related to poor perfusion among patients with idiopathic pulmonary fibrosis? Presented at the *Biannual Meeting of the Society of Respiratory Care Physicians...*

Why is such behavior lamentable? Because it is fundamentally *dishonest*. The number of abstracts should be dictated by the number of different research questions, not by the number of investigators wanting to be a first author. Although this may not seem like a major issue when abstracts are being prepared, it is likely to become important when the manuscript is written. Unless an abstract can stand alone as a distinct contribution, it will not stand alone as a manuscript. There is also the potential conflict over who will be the first author of the lone paper that these three abstracts can support. Do not count on Dr. Bigshot, the senior author, to help you sort this out. He is the culprit in the first place, for failing to exert his role as senior investigator to prevent multiple submissions of the same material. It is much better to clarify the list and order of authors at the very beginning, when basic decisions about abstracts are being made (see Chapter 10 on authorship).

What about submitting the same abstract twice or submitting two similar ones? Most meetings have rules concerning duplicate presentations. As long as the results have not been published as a manuscript, you are usually allowed to submit similar information a second time if the second meeting is "bigger" than the first meeting. In other words, if you have presented the results at a local or regional meeting, you can submit them to a national meeting; if they have been presented at a national meeting, they can be submitted to an international meeting. However, do this judiciously. Listing the same abstract several times in your CV is not a good idea; nor will an audience of scientists appreciate hearing about the same results twice. You are usually better off spending the time working on the manuscript than traveling to several scientific meetings to present and re-present the same results.

GETTING STARTED ON A MEETING ABSTRACT

In the simplest form, an abstract comprises four parts: (1) a sentence or two of *introduction,* (2) the essential aspects of the study's *methods,* (3) the main *results* of the study, and (4) a brief statement of your *conclusions* about the meaning of the study (each of these four sections is discussed in more detail in Chapters 3, 4, 5, and 8). In all sections, brevity is essential. It is often helpful to write the parts separately and then string them together at the end. Occasionally, a meeting requires that you submit a structured abstract, following specific rules on content and form.

Introduction

An introduction has one purpose: explaining why it was important to do the study. The introduction presents what is known and not known about the research topic. Sometimes, this part of an abstract is called the *background.* Do not make the common mistake of assuming that the answer is obvious. Just because you have spent a few years working on a problem does not mean that a reviewer or reader will be nearly as knowledgeable. Sometimes, stating the limitations of previous studies or beliefs helps: "Although many family practitioners believe they spend more time with depressed patients than internists do, this has never been evaluated in actual practice."

The introduction should be written in plain English, without jargon, run-on sentences, abbreviations, or acronyms. You want to make it as easy as possible for the reviewer to read on. The introduction usually ends with a one-sentence description of the research question, in the form of the study's objective. Examples are provided in Chapter 3.

Methods

The Methods section of the abstract should describe the study design, who was studied, what you measured, and how you analyzed the data. If it matters, you should mention where the subjects came from and how they were selected. Specify the number of subjects, by group if appropriate. All important measurement techniques should be described. You can leave out obvious methods (e.g., "subjects were asked their age and sex") as well as intricate details, unless they absolutely matter.

Results

Make sure you emphasize the main finding of the study. Concentrate on various aspects of that single result, such as the effects of adjusting for potential confounders, of using alternative definitions, or of looking for dose–response effects. It is better to be thorough about one result than attempt to present many unrelated findings. For example, suppose you find that hypertensive patients who take calcium channel blockers are more likely to have hemorrhagic strokes. It is more important to present your results by type of calcium channel blocker (long-acting vs. short-acting) and by type of bleed (subarachnoid vs. post-thrombotic) and to show that patients taking other antihypertensive medications did not have an increased risk than to present extraneous data with small P values, such as the finding that "patients who took diuretic medications had more gallstones ($P < 0.01$)."

Do not just present P values, F statistics, or regression coefficients. Make sure your effect size is clear (see Chapter 5 if you do not know the definition of an effect size). State your key results in words, followed by the numbers. For example, "Patients treated with cementamycin were nearly twice as likely to require dialysis as those treated with other aminoglycosides (20% vs. 11%; RR = 1.9; 95% CI = 1.3 to 2.8)." Use confidence intervals, or P values, to establish the precision and statistical significance of your findings (all these terms are discussed in Chapter 5).

Conclusions

What do you think your results mean? Be specific. Do not repeat the results in slightly different words or make silly declarations such as "These results may have clinical importance," "Our results should be confirmed by other investigators," "Our findings support our hypothesis," or "Further research is needed." Make a reasonable statement about the implications of your results. If the results have, or may have, clinical meaning, then say how. If another study is needed, then state what sort of study it should be. One quick test: If you could have written your conclusion before you knew your results, then you have not really concluded anything. Start over.

THE ABSTRACT SUBMISSION AND REVIEW PROCESS

Knowing how the review process works will help you prepare a better abstract as well as one that is more likely to be accepted for a meeting. First, it is imperative that you follow all the rules. Often, abstracts are processed by a company hired for this task, with employees who take their jobs seriously. Abstracts must be submitted on time to the correct address, and if a form is provided, the abstract must meet any size requirements. Take the instructions seriously. If the directions say 12-point font, or no more than 10 characters to the inch, they mean it. If a box is provided, stay within the lines. The same is true for the abstract deadline, as an hour late may be too late. Finally, you must include the appropriate fees and sign the form. So if a meeting does not accept credit cards, bring your checkbook to work on the day you plan to submit an abstract.

Abstracts are usually submitted to a single address, where they are registered and screened for adherence to all the rules. Only then are they dispersed for review. Most abstract forms have little check boxes that indicate the general topic area or methodology. These are used to determine which panel of scientists will be reviewing your abstract, so pay attention to them. You may be able to aim your abstract at a more sympathetic or appropriate group of reviewers this way. Often, it helps to ask a more senior investigator in the field for some advice. You may learn, for example, that one particular topic area (say, clinical epidemiology) tends to attract the toughest reviewers and the most abstracts at a particular meeting, whereas another (say, access to care) is often undersubscribed. Choosing a less popular area will not work, however, if the organizers of the meeting have decided to accept the same proportion of abstracts in each area. If a meeting has a scientific theme, and your research fits that theme, then take advantage of that because the meeting organizers will be looking for abstracts in that area.

Some meetings, especially international ones, may accept all, or nearly all, the abstracts submitted. In general, the higher the registration fee, the more likely an abstract will be accepted. For many groups, the annual or biennial meeting is a big money-making opportunity, particularly if there is extensive corporate sponsorship. That is why membership in the meeting's sponsoring organization is often a prerequisite for submission of an abstract. The more abstracts submitted, the more scientists who need to join the society; the more abstracts accepted, the more scientists who will pay the registration fee, attend the meeting, and be available to corporate representatives.

How Can I Make Sure That My Abstract Stands Out?

A review panel usually comprises between 3 and 10 reviewers, each of whom may receive 50 to 100, or sometimes more, abstracts to review. As a result, reviewers can spend only a few minutes with each abstract. They are looking for abstracts that seem to belong at the meeting, such as those with hot topics, large sample sizes, or impressive statistics. In their haste, reviewers may not notice subtly elegant design features or novel methodologic approaches unless you point them out. If your abstract has one of these attributes, say so:

> Although many have advocated ..., this has never been done. We therefore performed the first....

> To avoid these problems, we developed a new methodology that....

Reviewers may miss important results, especially if they are written in jargon. Use plain English to emphasize them:

> *Change:*

> In multivariable logistic regression analyses, there was a statistically significant linear association between serum HDL cholesterol levels measured in stored serum samples obtained at the time of enrollment and the odds of being diagnosed with an aortic aneurysm ($P < 0.001$) during follow-up.

To:

HDL cholesterol was an independent risk factor for aortic vascular disease, such that subjects with serum levels <35 mg/dL had three times (95% CI: 1.3 to 7) the risk of developing an aortic aneurysm than those with levels >55 mg/dL.

WHY ABSTRACTS ARE REJECTED

Reviewers look for reasons to reject an abstract, in part because it is usually easier to identify obviously bad work than to select really good work. But reviewers will usually not have time to notice subtle examples of bias or confounding, or your failure to use the most stringent statistical tests. That is why some highly rated abstracts turn out to be disappointing manuscripts: The additional details reveal previously unapparent flaws.

But some flaws are easy to spot, and usually lead to quick rejection of an abstract.

Dull Topic with Lots of Previous Research. Reviewers are almost always asked to judge an abstract's originality. You must include something new, or carefully specify how what you did is better than previous work. If your work is strictly confirmatory, then indicate why the confirmation was needed—for example, because only one or two studies had been done, or because the previous results were considered controversial.

No Context for the Research. Never assume that the reviewers will be sufficiently familiar with your specific field of research to understand why it is important. Take one or two sentences at the beginning of the abstract to explain the background for the work, and take another sentence at the end to discuss the implications of your results.

Small Number of Subjects. Limited sample size is especially problematic if the results are nonsignificant. Remember, reviewers are looking for a reason to reject, and a study of only 5 or even 20 patients is an invitation to do so. All is not lost, however, if your observation about those patients has earth-shattering importance. However, you will have to acknowledge the small sample and discuss why the research matters anyway.

No Numbers, All Talk. Most reviewers respond unfavorably to an abstract devoid of numbers, in part because it is not possible to tell whether the investigators studied one subject or 500, or whether they found anything of value. In some cases, abstracts lacking statistics fall in the same category. Numbers and statistics may not matter in your particular case (say, discovering a genetic defect that causes a rare disease), but in most cases, an anumeric abstract will face an uphill battle.

All Numbers, No Words. Abstracts crammed with lists of numbers with no clear explanation are often rejected. Reviewers do not have the time to figure out what an abstract might have said had the authors made it interpretable. Moreover, any important results will get drowned out by the noise.

Too Short. This may seem silly, but an abstract that is much shorter than all the other submissions may not be accepted. It will look strange. Fill—or at least come close to filling—the box or the allocated number of words.

Sloppiness. As with any submission, sloppiness in presentation will be interpreted—and should be interpreted—as a cause for concern about the general quality of the work. Check for typographical errors, simple arithmetical mistakes, and misspelled names. Read the abstract aloud to someone else.

Looks Too Different from Other Abstracts.   Find a copy of the previous year's abstracts, which are usually published as a journal supplement. Then compare the plenary abstracts with what you plan to submit. For example, were figures and tables used? What sort of research questions seemed to be in favor?

Phrases That Invite Rejection.   There are two phrases that will almost always result in your abstract being rejected: "Data will be presented" and "Results will be discussed." Never include either of these phrases in an abstract unless you have been invited to make a presentation at the meeting and were asked to submit an abstract by the meeting organizers.

Too Many Abbreviations, Too Much Data.   Lots of abbreviations and numbers may create the impression that you have done some real work, so your abstract may be less likely to be rejected outright. But they also make it harder for the reviewer to figure out whether you have done anything exceptional, so the likelihood of getting a high rating is also diminished. Demonstrating to a reviewer that you have many results is not nearly as important as showing that you have one important result that merits an oral or plenary presentation.

Ten or Twenty P Values.   An abstract that is full of P values is usually an abstract that lacks focus and effect sizes. Change a sentence such as "We found that fair skin ($P < 0.05$), sun exposure ($P < 0.01$), lack of use of sunscreen ($P < 0.001$), and residence in a beach community ($P < 0.0001$) were independently associated with skin cancer" into one that tells the reader what you found, and the strength of the association between each of these characteristics and skin cancer: "We identified several independent risk factors for skin cancer: fair skin (odds ratio [OR] = 1.6; 95% confidence interval [CI]: 1.0 to 2.6), failure to use sunscreen (OR = 2.0; CI: 1.4 to 2.9), and living in a beach community (RR = 5.0; CI: 2.0 to 12). Each hour of sun exposure per day increased the risk of skin cancer by 35% (95% CI: 10% to 66%)." The extra length leads to much greater clarity.

Overuse of "Respectively."   It is tempting to save space by listing variables, then the results followed by the word *respectively:* "The risks of glaucoma in White men, Black men, Asian men, White women, Black women, and Asian women were 8%, 12%, 6%, 4%, 6%, and 3%, respectively." This phrasing slows down and confuses the reader, who is forced to scan back and forth between the text and the numbers to figure out which ones go together, and then figure out if there is any sort of pattern. Reread the sentence in question, and you will see what I mean. Instead of using "respectively," rephrase the sentence to keep the groups and the percentages together, and to provide some interpretation of the results: "Glaucoma was more common in men than women and in blacks than in other racial groups. The risks in men were 8% in Whites, 12% in Blacks, and 6% in Asians; in women, they were 4% in Whites, 6% in Blacks, and 3% in Asians."

FITTING AN ABSTRACT INTO ITS SPACE

Nearly all meetings require that your abstract fits into a box of a predetermined size, or not exceed a certain word or character limit. If you have never had to fit an abstract into a limited space, you are probably wondering why this warrants an entire section in this chapter. Those who have already faced this problem know that this can be one of the most stressful aspects of writing an abstract.

Never leave the space-fitting process for the last minute. It is frustrating to have an abstract deadline in 10 minutes, only to discover that your abstract is not close to fitting. Do not drive your administrative assistant or research staff (or yourself) crazy trying to figure out a way to shorten your abstract. Plan in advance.

Begin by making an assessment of how far you have to go. Do you have an extra line or two, or is the abstract almost twice as long as permissible? Abstracts that need only minor shortening are a snap. Work directly from a single-spaced copy that almost fits. Look for lines with only a few words: It is almost always possible to trim a few words from one of the preceding sentences in the paragraph, thus shortening the abstract by a full line. Sometimes, the title is a word or two too long, so that it runs onto an extra line. Does the list of institutions involved in the research take up too much room? Can it be abbreviated?

Change:

Effects of mathematics and science education on subsequent career choices of high school students. Rosen A, Greenstein S, Sforza J, University of New York at Franklin Square, Franklin Square, NY.

To:

Math and science education and career choices of high school students. Rosen A, Greenstein S, Sforza J, Univ. of New York at Franklin Square.

Eliminate descriptive words (e.g., very, quite, even, highly, strongly) and introductory phrases (e.g., we found that, our results demonstrate that). Look for nouns that can be made into verbs:

Change:

In order to accurately measure vitamin C levels in subjects' serum, we used a modification of the Storey technique.

To:

We measured serum vitamin C levels by modifying the Storey technique.

Change:

We conclude that bilirubin levels are more useful in determining the prognosis of patients who have cirrhosis due to alcoholic liver disease than they are in patients who have cirrhosis due to chronic viral hepatitis.

To:

Bilirubin levels are more useful in determining prognosis in patients with cirrhosis because of alcoholic liver disease than in those with cirrhosis because of chronic viral hepatitis.

Look for sentences that can be combined:

Change:

We enrolled 124 subjects with rheumatoid arthritis from the rheumatology clinic. They were randomly assigned to an intervention group ($n = 63$) or a control group ($n = 61$).

To:

> Rheumatoid arthritis patients followed in the rheumatology clinic were randomly assigned to an intervention ($n = 63$) or control group ($n = 61$).

Check for words that can be hyphenated. Many word-processing programs can hyphenate text automatically. Delete unneeded spaces; note that word-processed (as opposed to typed) documents need only one space following a period. Finally, look for unnecessary abbreviations. Did you use an abbreviation in the first sentence but never again in the rest of the abstract?

What If You Are Still Not Close?

If your abstract is still too long, or if you know from the start that it will require major surgery, you will need a different approach. Deleting a word here or there will not suffice. Begin by printing a double-spaced version of the abstract. This will make the abstract look a lot longer and remind you of how much information you have included. Delete anything that does not convey the meaning of the abstract. It is tempting to present interesting results that are a little off the topic, or methodologic niceties, but they will need to be sacrificed. Be merciless. Leave out measurement methods if there are no associated results. Delete results if they are irrelevant to your conclusions. Look for similar phrases that appear several times in separate sentences, then link the sentences:

Change:

> Compared with women, men were twice as likely to bicycle for exercise. This difference was statistically significant at $P < 0.01$. Compared with men, women were 1.5 times more likely to walk for exercise. This difference was also statistically significant at $P < 0.02$.

To:

> Men were twice as likely as women to bicycle for exercise ($P < 0.01$), whereas women were 1.5 times more likely to walk ($P < 0.02$).

If you will be presenting many such comparisons, then indicate in the methods section that "exercise rates in men and women were compared as relative risks (RR) with 95% confidence intervals." Then you can say in the results section:

> Men were more likely to bicycle (RR = 2.0; 1.2 to 3.6); women were more likely to walk (RR = 1.5; 1.2 to 2.1).

Consider summarizing your results in a table or figure, if allowed. This can save a lot of space if you have to repeat the same type of results more than three or four times. Often, you can convert a background of two or three sentences into a single introductory phrase:

Change:

> Some previous studies have found that exposure to sunlight in infancy is associated with the subsequent development of melanoma. Other studies have not confirmed this effect. We prospectively studied....

To:

To determine whether exposure to sunlight in infancy is associated with the development of melanoma, we prospectively studied....

Change:

The testosterone receptor has three common phenotypes, designated TT, Tt, and tt. The tt phenotype may be more common among subjects with coronary artery disease. We studied....

To:

To determine whether the tt phenotype of the testosterone receptor is associated with coronary artery disease, we studied....

Sometimes, you can save space in an abstract by indicating the measurement or analytic methodology in a sentence containing study results.

Change:

Diabetes was assessed by self-report. ... Differences between groups were compared using the chi-squared statistic. ... Diabetic subjects were three times as likely to have gallstones ($P < 0.01$).

To:

Patients with self-reported diabetes were three times as likely to have gallstones ($P < 0.01$ by chi-squared test).

Finally, unless the rules require it, do not right-justify (full-justify) the margins of your abstract. Such text is harder to read and may take up more space.

ABSTRACTS FOR MANUSCRIPTS

The purpose of the abstract that accompanies a manuscript is straightforward: to present the basic substance of the study and to entice the reader (and the reviewer) to read the manuscript. Keep it simple.

The commonest mistakes are reusing the same abstract that you submitted to a meeting and using an abstract that is unnecessarily complicated. If your manuscript is accepted, almost everyone who reads your abstract will have access to the full-length article; after all, it has been published. The same is true in the manuscript review process. Even if someone is reading the abstract on the Internet, that person will either have access to a medical library or can contact you for a reprint.

Minor details should be omitted from the abstract (but most should be included in the text, of course). For example, seldom is it necessary to mention the number of subjects with missing data or the exact recruitment period. There is seldom a need to describe your subjects in great detail (e.g., the age, sex, and race distribution) or to explain complicated findings. These are the reasons why the abstract for a paper is sometimes more appropriately called a summary.

Many journals now require that authors submit a structured abstract, with specific sections dictated by each journal's rules. Imposing a uniform framework ensures that all the key points are covered. Structured abstracts are just like ordinary abstracts, with one exception: They are rarely written in complete sentences. The basic parts—Background, Methods, Results, and Conclusions—remain, although some may be further divided into subsections.

   A sample abstract follows. If you are having a hard time getting going, start with the sample (or another abstract that you have admired), and make changes as appropriate for your own study.

Is Sliced Bread All It Is Cracked Up to Be? A Randomized Controlled Trial

Background Although it is commonly believed that sliced bread was a great invention, there are no firm data establishing that it represents an improvement over intact loaves. We performed a randomized trial to determine whether people really do prefer sliced bread.

Methods One thousand bread-consuming volunteer families, consisting of three or more persons between the age of 2 and 75 years living in the San Francisco area, were randomly allocated to receive either sliced bread ($n = 503$) or intact loaves ($n = 497$) for 1 year. A choice of breads (including sourdough and cracked wheat) was delivered free, daily. Bread was radiolabeled with yeast[75] to facilitate blinded measurement of the amount discarded in the trash. We measured happiness with bread on a 1 (least happy) to 7 (happiest) scale with the Muffinburger questionnaire. Bread preference, as weekly consumption (kg delivered minus kg discarded), was estimated. Mean consumption and happiness per group, and the mean difference between the groups (sliced-loaf minus intact-loaf), with 95% confidence intervals, were determined.

Results Consumption of bread was similar in the two groups: The mean difference was 0.1 (–0.1 to 0.3) kg. Families in the sliced-bread group consumed 1.2 (0.9 to 1.5) kg per week, whereas those in the intact-loaf group ate 1.3 (0.8 to 1.8) kg per week. More families in the intact-loaf group than in the sliced-bread group consumed 2 kg or more of bread per week (34% vs. 26%; $P < 0.01$ by chi-squared test), but fewer families in the sliced-bread group ate no bread at all (3% vs. 8% in the intact-loaf group; $P < 0.002$). Bread happiness was similar in the two groups: 3.5 (3.0 to 4.0) in the sliced-bread group, and 3.7 (3.0 to 4.4) in the intact-loaf group.

Conclusions The use of sliced bread as a gold standard, as well as other clichés, needs to be reevaluated.

Even that abstract can be trimmed if necessary; here is a shorter version:

Is Sliced Bread All It Is Cracked Up to Be?
A Randomized Controlled Trial

There are no firm data establishing that sliced bread represents an improvement over intact loaves. We performed a randomized trial to determine bread preference in 1,000 bread-consuming families who were randomly allocated to receive either sliced bread ($n = 503$) or intact loaves ($n = 497$) delivered free, daily for 1 year. Bread was radiolabeled with yeast[75] to facilitate blinded measurement of the amount discarded. Consumption of bread was similar in the two groups ($P = 0.54$): Families in the sliced-bread group consumed 1.2 (95% confidence interval: 0.9 to 1.5) kg per week, whereas those in the intact-loaf group ate 1.3 (0.8 to 1.8) kg per week. More families in the intact-loaf group than in the sliced-bread group consumed 2 kg or more of bread per week (34% vs. 26%; $P < 0.01$), but fewer in the sliced-bread group (3%) ate no bread at all (vs. 8%; $P < 0.002$). Bread happiness on the Muffinburger scale was similar in the two groups. The use of sliced bread as a gold standard as well other clichés needs to be reevaluated.

✔ CHECKLIST FOR

TITLE AND ABSTRACT

Title

1. Are the title and the research question closely related?

2. Is the title objective in tone?

3. Are special features of the study mentioned?

Abstract

1. Are there introduction, methods, results, and conclusions sections, even if not explicitly labeled as such?

2. Are the five or six main features of the study mentioned?

3. Are the key results of the study stated in words?

4. Do the conclusions follow from the results? Do they make a meaningful statement?

5. Did you follow all the rules of the meeting or the journal?

Reference

1. Hulley SB, Cummings SR, Browner WS, et al., eds. *Designing Clinical Research: An Epidemiologic Approach*. 3rd ed. Philadelphia, PA: Lippincott Williams & Wilkins; 2007.

3 Introduction

The introduction to a manuscript has two main purposes: to entice readers to look further and then to tell them what to expect. In addition, during the manuscript review stage, the introduction must also demonstrate to reviewers that they are reading the work of a professional. Sometimes a well-written abstract can serve this role, but many reviewers will begin by reading a paper's introduction. Make sure that you do not disappoint them. Even better, use the introduction to show reviewers how thoroughly you understand the field, how clearly you think, and how well you write.

Almost every introduction should include four elements: (1) the background of the research question, (2) previous research in the area, (3) problems with that research, and (4) what you did to fix those problems. Each of these four elements warrants at least one sentence, but more than one paragraph per element is seldom needed. As a general rule, you should leave out any information that does not fit into one of these four categories. There are a few exceptions. The introduction to an article in some basic science journals includes an overview of the methods and a brief summary of the results of the study. For example, "In this paper, we show that hyperphosphatasia (Type IB) is caused by a point mutation in the 4-α-hydroxybutyl receptor." Some psychiatry and psychology journals expect much longer introductions, with an extensive review of the literature and current theories. Look at a few issues of the journal to which you plan to submit your manuscript and see how most introductions are formatted.

In contrast to the introduction to a full-length manuscript, the introduction to an abstract must establish only the background of the research: Why was the research question meaningful? All the other points are optional, although a one-sentence description of how you set out to answer the research question may be useful.

THE BACKGROUND OF THE RESEARCH QUESTION

Start the introduction with a few words about the overall topic of your research. The topic can be a disease (e.g., uterine cancer), a risk factor (e.g., exposure to asbestos), a therapy (e.g., cisplatin), a technique (e.g., magnetic resonance imaging), or a group of patients (e.g., Hispanic women). Do not try to cover all these possibilities. Select the topic or topics that best reflect the unique contribution of your research.

Too Many Details:

Magnetic resonance spectroscopy of the pelvis may have the capability to identify responders to cisplatin among Hispanic women with cervical cancer owing to herpes virus infection.

Focused on the Topic:

Magnetic resonance spectroscopy may identify which patients with cancer are most responsive to therapy.

Leaving out some of the details (such as the type of cancer and the exact therapy) helps orient the reader to expect a manuscript that focuses on the utility of a specific diagnostic test.

Avoid triviality. Tell the reader something *new,* or tell it in a novel way. An intriguing first sentence will be worth the extra work.

Trivial (Is There Anyone Who Does Not Already Know This?):

Pulmonary artery catheters are often used in critically ill patients.

Informative:

Since their development more than 35 years ago, nearly 300 million pulmonary artery catheters have been used in the United States.

Another trap is the unessential fact that does not have anything to do with your research. It is better to intrigue the reader.

True, but Dull and Not Relevant to the Topic:

Stomach cancer is now the 15th leading cause of cancer in the United States.

Intriguing:

The incidence of stomach cancer has declined by almost 80% in the United States since the 1930s.

Unless you are writing for a specialized audience, you need to provide some context. Do not just launch into your exposition.

Arcane:

The risk of cirrhosis among compound heterozygotes (cys282/his63) for the *HFE* gene is not certain.

This topic statement might be adequate for an article in the *Journal of Hemochromatosis Genetics* (if there were such a journal). But if you send your manuscript to a less-specialized journal, only those readers who remember the common mutations that cause hemochromatosis will be able to continue. So a better idea would be to write a few sentences explaining each of these terms.

Reader-Friendly:

Hemochromatosis is an inherited disorder that manifests as diabetes, bronze discoloration of the skin, and liver disease. The two commonest genetic defects involve mutations (cys282 and his63) in the *HFE* gene. The risk of cirrhosis in a

compound heterozygote (someone who has one copy of each of these two mutations) is not known.

Notice how the "reader-friendly" example provides the knowledge needed to read
the paper and may even persuade someone to continue.

PREVIOUS RESEARCH IN THE AREA

The section on existing research flows logically from the background of the problem, as you move from the general to the specific. You do not need to provide a
complete literature review. Provide a synthetic summary of what is known, rather
than a boring list of every previous study.

> ### Pedantic (Albeit All-Too-Common):
>
> There have been six previous studies in this area. Sanford, in a study of 341 pa-
> tients from Great Britain, found.... Bannister, studying 45 patients in Milwaukee,
> showed.... Ward followed 211 patients, and found....

> ### Synthetic:
>
> Previous studies in this area have had conflicting results, some suggesting that...,
> whereas others found that....

Even if you had already done a thorough literature search when you started your
study, do not forget to update it when you write the manuscript. If you have not done
a literature review before you started your research project, you may be in for a rude
awakening when you discover that another researcher, and perhaps many others,
have already done your study. If you are not familiar with how to do computerized
literature searches, get some assistance from a medical librarian. Be sure to go back
at least 15 (or even 20) years and to read the text of any relevant articles, not just
their abstracts. Your manuscript is probably going to be reviewed by several experts,
few of whom will show mercy if you are not thoroughly familiar with the literature.

If there is no research in the area, explain why. Discuss existing beliefs and
where they may have originated.

> Despite the obvious importance of this question, there are no controlled studies
> of the use of mentholated skin creams for upper respiratory infections. Current
> practice apparently reflects a consensus among grandparents of its efficacy.

How Do I Decide What Studies to Cite?

Sometimes there are one or two "seminal articles" in a field, by which I mean
those that either opened the area for research or provided information that has
changed clinical practice or scientific knowledge. Those studies should always be
cited, sometimes even mentioning the first author by name. If there is a recent (and
thorough) review article, that is also worth citing. You will also have the opportunity
to reference specific studies in the next section of the introduction, where you point
out some of the limitations of previous research. Seldom is it necessary to list more
than 10 articles in the introduction.

Cite studies in chronologic order, beginning with the oldest one. It is a nice touch that shows that you have paid attention to the history of how knowledge was acquired in the field.

PROBLEMS WITH PAST RESEARCH

After discussing what past researchers have done, you need to explain why you did your study. Specify the problems with the existing research in the area. Perhaps previous studies did not follow subjects long enough or used the wrong design. Subjects may have been selected so carefully that the results of those studies do not apply in practice, or are not selected carefully enough, so that no one is really sure whether the diagnoses were correct. Previous researchers may have used poor measurement techniques or an inadequate analysis. Various design flaws may have introduced bias.

That previous studies were imperfect may not provide a sufficient rationale for your study. For example, suppose previous researchers failed to use the latest measurement technique; by itself, this does not matter. But if they failed to find an effect, or if the previous methods were faulty and would lead to erroneous conclusions, that would matter. Explain this.

Uninformative:

No prior study has used the newly developed supersensitive radioimmunoassay to measure serum porcelain titers.

Explanatory:

Because previous investigators did not use the recently developed supersensitive radioimmunoassay, their studies may have failed to detect an association between serum porcelain titers and palindromic fibromyalgia.

Be careful not to criticize a study unless your work represents an improvement. In some cases, previous studies are pretty good, perhaps even better than your own research. Do not create a problem where one does not exist.

Silly:

Although there have been more than 20 well-done randomized trials of coronary stenting for acute myocardial infarction, no previous study was written by a second-year cardiology fellow in her spare time.

Relevant:

Previous studies of stenting in acute myocardial infarction have not determined the practicality of the therapy in the developing world.

Sometimes, you or a colleague may have done the most relevant prior studies. In these situations, you should explain why you also did the current study. Make it obvious when you cite previous work from your research group, rather than making believe that "Smith" (assuming that's your name) is someone else.

Misleading:

A prior study by Adams, Williams, and Maxwell had an average follow-up of only 1 month.

True:

We previously reported survival at 1 month in these subjects.

Do not be hypercritical or overly detailed in your criticism. Your reviewer may be a colleague of the lambasted author who uses the same methodology. Worse, the reviewer may be the subject of your criticism herself. Instead, describe the general category of the problem. Avoid antagonistic phrases (e.g., "failed to," "made the mistake of," "used invalid techniques") and singling out a specific author for blame.

Harsh:

Incredibly, Langford—an incompetent researcher if there ever was one, despite his Nobel Prize and an endowed chair at Harvard—did not recognize the importance of asking about prior history of stroke, and erroneously misclassified several living subjects as dead because they did not return a questionnaire.

Gentle:

Previous research did not account for the possible effects of a history of stroke or have 100% complete follow-up.

Even better, sometimes you can cite another author who has criticized the prior study in an editorial, review, or letter to the editor. The use of the passive voice softens the blow:

The results of that study have been questioned because …

Some have suggested that the results of this study can be interpreted as showing that …

Sometimes, there is nothing wrong with previous research: Some studies found black, and others found white. If that is the case, then say so, providing the references.

Of the three previous studies of this question, two found that a routine program of physical therapy for elderly inpatients was associated with a modest reduction in length of hospital stay (4, 5), whereas another study concluded that there was no benefit (6).

 ## WHAT YOU DID TO FIX THOSE PROBLEMS

Conclude the introduction by telling the reader about the major improvements you have made on past research. Here is your chance to highlight innovative features of your design, sample, or measurement methods. The introduction should end with a one-sentence overview of your study:

To address these problems, we documented variceal bleeding using a newly developed noninvasive in situ scintigraphic technique. Patients who were bleeding at a rate of 20 mL/minute or more were randomly assigned to sclerotherapy with either SuperGlue or shark liver oil, and followed for rebleeding, length of hospital stay, and 6-month mortality.

If your study is a "sequel" to a prior study from your research group, clearly state how the current study expands on that work. Are you reanalyzing previously reported data? Did you enroll new or additional subjects? Did you develop a new methodology? Have the results changed because of additional follow-up? Reviewers are often skeptical about manuscripts that appear to "re-report" old data, so it is essential to highlight the new stuff:

> We expand our prior findings by including 50 additional patients, for a total of 96, as well as the results of the newly developed latex heterophile agglomeration test.

Finally, edit your introduction and remove whatever is not necessary. See Chapter 14 for some tips.

✔ CHECKLIST FOR

INTRODUCTION

1. Are the four major elements of the manuscript introduction (background, existing research, problems with that research, and your improvements) covered in four or fewer paragraphs?

2. After reading the introduction, was someone not familiar with the field able to tell why you did the study, and how your study is an improvement over existing knowledge?

3. Do you use an objective tone when criticizing previous work?

4. Do you describe how your study addresses the problems of previous research?

5. Is there anything extraneous in your introduction?

4 ◆ Methods

The Methods section of a manuscript is usually the easiest part to write, so if you are having a difficult time getting going, it is a good place to start. The section has four straightforward purposes: to tell readers what type of study you did (*design*), whom or what you studied (*subjects*), what you measured (*measurements*), and how you analyzed the data (*analysis*). A successful Methods section provides enough detail so that knowledgeable readers will understand how you did your study, and other investigators could reproduce your study (or the part they are interested in).

But many novice investigators lose sight of the methods forest for the methods twigs. They are so concerned with getting every detail correct that it is impossible to discern the overall plan of the study. If you have not already done so at the end of the introduction, start the Methods section by providing an overall description of the study in a sentence or two (e.g., "We performed a case–control study of the risk factors for chronic lymphocytic leukemia in textile workers."). Then begin each subsection with one or two sentences of description that orient the reader to the general subtopic (e.g., subjects, measurements).

The Results section and the Methods section of a manuscript are linked inextricably. If you mention something in the results, then you must describe how you measured it in the methods. Similarly, if you describe how you measured something in the methods, you should present the results of that measurement. These rules imply that every item in the Methods section should have an isomorph in the results and vice versa.

As with any part of the manuscript, if you are having a difficult time getting started, begin by writing a simple description. You can elaborate later. Indeed, a "keep it simple" approach is valuable to provide a clear framework for the Methods section even if you are not having trouble.

We studied whether a new drug would make people with headaches feel better than they did if they took aspirin. We asked lots of people who had frequent headaches whether they wanted to be in the study. If they said yes, and if they were in good health, we flipped a coin to see if they would get to take the new pill or aspirin. We made the pills look identical so that no one could tell them apart. We gave everybody two pills and told them to take the pills at the first symptom of a headache; an hour later, we asked them if their headache was better. We compared the percentage of patients in each group who said that their headache was completely or almost completely gone.

DESIGN

Most, but not all, studies fit neatly into one of the main types of research designs: case series, cross-sectional study, case–control study, cohort study, before–after study, or a clinical trial. Some studies incorporate more than one design. For example, a cross-sectional study of the frequency of alcohol abuse in a methadone clinic might be followed by a prospective cohort study of the subjects with alcoholism who had been identified. In this sort of situation, both designs should be mentioned.

> We performed a cross-sectional study of the prevalence of alcohol abuse among patients cared for in the general medical and family practice clinics and then prospectively followed those who were actively abusing alcohol.

If you are not sure what sort of design you used, it may be helpful to refer to Figure 4-1 or to review a few of the chapters in *Designing Clinical Research*.[1] (*Note:* The figure does not include studies of diagnostic or prognostic tests, or synthetic studies such as meta-analyses and decision analyses.)

Indicate whether the study was done prospectively (the subjects were followed as part of the study protocol) or retrospectively (follow-up, if any, occurred before the study started, as in most chart review studies). It is also important to mention whether the study was performed as a secondary data analysis, that is, an analysis of data collected for a different purpose than your study. This tells readers and reviewers why data that were not part of the initial aims of the study may not have been collected. Be explicit about the limitations that this type of design may have introduced:

> We performed a secondary data analysis of the predictors of estrogen replacement therapy among women enrolled in a multicenter study of the efficacy of glucose control in patients with stroke. Therefore, data on the exact estrogen preparations used were not available.

Avoid having an overly detailed single-sentence description of the design; it will just confuse readers. Even if you performed a prospective, run-in, randomized, double-blind, double dummy, placebo-controlled, parallel group, 16-week study (yes, this a real design!), just call it a randomized trial or a randomized double-blind trial. The other details can be mentioned later. (Indeed, as retrospective trials are almost unheard of, do not include the word "prospective" in the description of a randomized trial.)

If applicable, mention key features of the design, such as random assignment or blinding:

> Subjects and investigators were blinded to group assignment and followed for at least 6 months.

> We performed a random-digit telephone survey in the Cleveland metropolitan area.

> We used a case–control design in which patients with acute leukemia were compared with two control groups: patients with solid tumors and those admitted for orthopedic procedures.

Do not say that you studied a "database." Instead, mention why patients were included in the database:

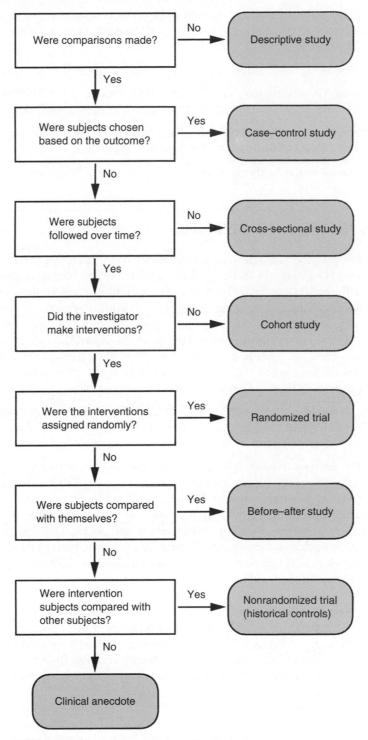

FIGURE 4-1. A rough guide to research designs

> We reviewed the medical records of Medicare patients in the state of California who had a discharge diagnosis of sepsis following a computerized review of 2009 billing records.

The design of a simple study can be mentioned at the end of the introduction:

> We performed a case–control study of the factors associated with a favorable prognosis among patients with documented influenza infection.

> We enrolled a cohort of patients with gastroesophageal reflux disease, who were subsequently followed for an average of 2 years.

In this situation, the Methods section can begin with a description of the subjects.

SUBJECTS AND SETTING

You must provide enough information about where you did your study and how you chose your subjects so that readers can determine to whom the results of the study will apply. Distinguish between your sampling plans (e.g., a random sample of residents of Chicago between the ages of 40 and 64 years) and the actual sample (those who responded to a newspaper advertisement for volunteers).

Do not be coy about the setting for a study by referring vaguely to "an academic medical center" or "a public hospital." Anyone reading the study will be able to tell, simply by looking at the authors' addresses, where the study took place. You might as well provide a brief description of the hospital or clinic.

> We enrolled patients with a diagnosis of hepatocellular carcinoma seen from 2008 to 2010 at the California Pacific Medical Center, a 600-bed hospital in San Francisco.

(*Note:* For reasons that are not clear, some journals prefer that you do not mention the specific site of your study, especially in the abstract. If this is the case, the journal editors will let you know during the manuscript review process.)

Readers and reviewers will want to know whether your subjects are representative of other subjects or patients with similar conditions. Did you enroll every patient with scleroderma in a medical clinic or just those with certain characteristics? What sort of medical clinic was it? Were your subjects volunteers who answered an advertisement in the local newspaper, or were they recruited from a subspecialist's practice?

Pay special attention to critical factors that reviewers and readers will want to know. For example, in a study of patients with lower back pain, what criteria were used to make the diagnosis? Were there any exceptions? Were subjects selected from a university-affiliated neurosurgery clinic? Were *prevalent* (previously diagnosed) or *incident* (newly diagnosed) cases enrolled? If prevalent cases were enrolled, how did you determine how long they had had back pain?

List your inclusion criteria (attributes that all subjects needed to have) and exclusion criteria (attributes that eliminated subjects from being eligible for the study). What specific qualifications did the subjects have to meet? These can range from relatively mundane characteristics, such as age, sex, race, and geographic location, to more complex attributes.

> We enrolled adults between ages 18 and 45 years who were members of a pre-paid health plan in Sacramento, CA, and who responded to a mailed request

for volunteers with a family history of asthma in a first-degree relative. Subjects were required to have no personal history of asthma or pulmonary disease, nor could they be taking any corticosteroids, bronchodilators, or β-blocker medications.

There is no clear distinction between inclusion and exclusion criteria, but saying that you enrolled only men seems somehow less offensive than saying that women were excluded.

What if your study was not very tightly designed, and you enrolled subjects with loose criteria on a haphazard basis, for example, as they showed up in the clinic on a day when you or a coinvestigator happened to be there? Then say so.

> We enrolled patients with shoulder pain of <4 weeks' duration who presented to our medical clinic when a coinvestigator was available.

> During a 6-month period, we enrolled a convenience sample of patients, including most of those who were admitted to the medical intensive care unit at our hospital during daytime hours on weekdays.

If you can, tell the reader how many of the potential subjects were actually enrolled in the study and why others were not enrolled.

> During the enrollment period (February 2008 to April 2010), 311 patients were admitted to the coronary care unit at Mills Peninsula Medical Center with a diagnosis of unstable angina or rule-out myocardial infarction; we enrolled 201 (65%) of these patients. Of the 110 patients we did not enroll, 46 were admitted after midnight, 23 did not speak English, and 11 died within 6 hours of admission. Twenty other patients were not enrolled for miscellaneous reasons; 10 patients refused to participate.

An alternative approach involves presenting enrollment data in the Results section. There are no absolute rules on which way is preferable.

Just as important as saying how many subjects were enrolled is telling the reader what happened to the subjects *after* they were enrolled. Few studies have complete data on all subjects; usually, at least a few drop out. Make sure to mention how you dealt with subjects who dropped out of the study. In which analyses, if any, were these subjects included?

> Of the 78 subjects initially enrolled, 5 refused follow-up; they have been excluded from all analyses.

> Of the 78 subjects initially enrolled, 5 refused follow-up; they have been excluded from analyses of quality-of-life outcomes.

Mention the time involved. If you recruited patients who were admitted to the hospital between January 1, 2009 and June 30, 2009, then say so, even if that information does not seem important at the time. Years later, it may matter if, for instance, treatments have changed or seasonal patterns are discovered.

Although this book is not written for preclinical scientists, the same concerns about subject and setting apply if your subjects are laboratory animals. Where did you get your rats? What species were they? Were they fed a special diet? How old were they? Did you impose any weight or activity restrictions? How many animals died before the experiment was completed? Incidentally, blinding also matters in animal research, although it is all too infrequent; indeed, cages are often labeled with the treatment that the "subject" received.

A few types of studies are subject to special rules. For instance, in a case–control study, there are two samples of subjects, the *cases* and the *controls*. They are described separately.

> Cases (n = 78) were selected from among patients admitted to the hospital with bleeding peptic ulcers, defined by gastroduodenoscopy. Controls (n = 183) were selected from among patients admitted to the psychiatry service.

If both the cases and the controls were selected from a larger group, then that group is described first.

> Cases and controls were selected from a cohort of graduate students in the social sciences at the University of Antwerp in 2007. Cases (n = 50) were those seen at the student health service who had one or more anxiety attacks during the ensuing year. Controls (n = 100) were randomly selected from among students who visited the same clinic to receive a mandatory flu shot.

If there were restrictions on how controls were selected—for instance, if controls were matched to cases on some criterion or criteria—these should also be mentioned.

> For each case, we selected two controls from among patients followed in the urology clinic; controls were matched for sex, age (within 3 years), and race (white, black, and others).

Explain how subjects were assigned to a group. If subjects were assigned randomly to alternative treatments, you should describe exactly how that was done. The most important question is whether it was possible to know the group a subject would be assigned to *before* he or she was enrolled in the study.

> After subjects were enrolled in the study, they were randomly assigned in approximately equal numbers, using a computer-generated random number table, to the intervention or control groups. An off-site programmer who was not involved in recruiting of patients made the assignments.

More details on special rules are provided later in this chapter under the heading "Special Situations."

You might wonder whether you should describe the people in your study as *subjects, patients,* or *participants* (it is easier with rodents—they are just called *mice, rats,* or *rabbits!*). Sometimes, the choice is clear.

> Subjects were volunteer medical students desperate for the $150 we paid them for undergoing three lumbar punctures and two right-sided heart catheterizations.

> Patients were a consecutive sample of those admitted to the intensive care unit with the diagnosis of sepsis.

At other times, the distinction between subjects and patients is less clear.

> Subjects were patients in the gastroenterology clinic who agreed to be participants in our study.

Studies involving people almost always require approval of a human subjects committee, and most such studies also require informed consent from the subjects. If this was the case in your study, you should so indicate. If not, mention why committee approval or subject consent was not needed.

MEASUREMENTS

What to Include?

Measurements should be presented in a logical order. It is most convenient to divide them into two groups: *predictor* variables (sometimes called *independent variables*) and *outcome variables* (sometimes called *dependent variables*).

Begin by describing how you measured the predictor variables. For example, did you review charts, ask patients to fill out a questionnaire, or interview them? Were medical diagnoses ascertained by patient self-report? Were they verified with medical records?

> We ascertained patients' demographic characteristics with a written questionnaire. Patients were specifically asked whether a physician had ever told them that they had hypertension, diabetes, or stroke. A history of heart disease was noted if a patient reported a previous myocardial infarction, coronary revascularization, or the use of nitroglycerine to treat exertional chest pain. We defined hypertension as either a history of physician-diagnosed high blood pressure, use of antihypertensive medications, or a systolic (diastolic) blood pressure >160 (90) mm Hg recorded on at least two occasions in the medical record.

Note that demographic is an adjective, not a noun, and it refers to basic attributes such as age, sex, and race, not medical history. Besides, there is no such thing as "demographics"—use demographic characteristics.

Develop an ordering system for how you present measurements of the predictor variables that you are comfortable with. The example below follows the standard order for presenting a patient at rounds: history, physical examination, and laboratory results.

History

General attributes (age, sex, and race)

Medical problems/history

Risk factors/habits

Family history

Medications

Education/socioeconomic status

Physical Exam

Height, weight

Vital signs

Other findings

Laboratory Results

Simple, routine studies

Specialized measurements

If your primary predictor variable (such as aspirin use) falls in the middle of a group, start a new paragraph for emphasis. Be sure to describe the measurement technique in adequate detail.

> We asked about use of medications, including aspirin (current, past 2 years, average weekly dose), in a nurse-administered interview.

If the study is a clinical trial, always include a separate paragraph describing the intervention and the control treatments in detail. If placebo tablets were used, could they be distinguished from the active pills? If you have not already done so in the section on subjects, it is helpful to begin that paragraph by describing how subjects were randomly assigned (not "randomized") to each group.

> Subjects were randomly assigned to either the intervention group or the control group. Group assignments were generated using a computer algorithm that allocated patients in approximately equal numbers to both groups. Assignments were sealed in numbered opaque envelopes that were opened after enrollment. The intervention group received 500 mg of panaceamycin three times daily (at 7 AM, 3 PM, and 10 PM) for 10 days; the control group was given identical placebo tablets.

After describing the predictor variables, mention how you measured the outcome variables. Begin by describing how you followed subjects, if it matters. For example, did you ascertain the occurrence of outcomes by periodic phone calls, return of prestamped postcards, follow-up clinic visits, or review of medical records? Next, discuss how you measured and handled the main outcome variable. Did you have a hierarchy of outcome variables, so that, for example, a subject with both an upper respiratory infection and pneumonia was counted as the more serious outcome of pneumonia? Or did you count whichever outcome occurred first?

> We followed patients for 30 days for the occurrence of pulmonary embolism. All patients were examined daily while hospitalized and telephoned weekly after discharge with inquiries about symptoms of dyspnea, pleuritic chest pain, hemoptysis, and leg swelling. If any of these were present, patients were evaluated according to a preset protocol that involved measurement of vital signs, oxygen saturation in room air, chest radiograms, electrocardiograms, D-dimers, and Doppler ultrasound examinations of the legs. Ventilation–perfusion scans were obtained for all patients who were judged by the study clinicians to have a 5% or greater chance of having a pulmonary embolism.

Finally, discuss secondary outcome variables, such as length of stay, hospital charges, or levels of various biochemical parameters.

At What Level of Detail?

Probably the most difficult aspect of writing about your measurements is determining the appropriate level of detail. Feel free to leave out methods if they are reasonably obvious (such as how you determined age or sex). You can make a global statement such as "We ascertained demographic characteristics by questionnaire (or chart review or phone interview)."

The level of detail must be appropriate for the intended audience. Always consider the technical sophistication of your readers and likely reviewers. Do not insult them. In a manuscript for the *Journal of Biochemistry,* you should not state that "the polymerase chain reaction was used to amplify DNA." In a paper likely to be reviewed by an epidemiologist or a biostatistician, you should not scrimp on the Analysis section by saying, "Data were analyzed using the DATANALYSIS software package." No matter how good your study, this sort of inattention leads reviewers to assume that you did not know what you were doing, and their review of your work will be less positive.

If you did something unusual, or used an unfamiliar or tricky method, tell the reader why you did it that way, and how you did it.

> To reduce the possibility of recall bias, we asked subjects a series of questions unrelated to our research hypothesis.

> Because this test may give false-positive results in the presence of active infection, we excluded patients who were febrile (>37.5°C) or who had been treated with antibiotics during the previous 2 weeks.

By explaining why, you head off reviewers' tendency to assume that if you did something in a nonstandard way, it was because the results would have been nonsignificant or unimportant if they had been obtained using more standard methods.

Provide greater detail about essential variables. In a study of the relation between cigarette smoking and dementia, you might mention that information on smoking, including current consumption, lifetime average consumption, age began smoking, and age quit smoking, was obtained by means of a validated questionnaire; you would also cite the appropriate reference.

Laboratory studies require a complete description of unique techniques. If a well-known technique was used, then say so, and cite the reference.

> We used the go-go-Niners method, except that we also cheered on first down.

Other techniques, if published in readily available literature, require less detailed descriptions. The basic rule applies: Provide enough detail to show that you are a competent scientist. In particular, challenging aspects of the procedure should be included.

> Maintaining a stable body weight in the mice required daily attention to diet, especially in the first 2 days following injection of cachexin.

Alternative techniques that were tried and discarded should be discussed.

> We considered using the low-light technique but had too difficult a time reading the fine print; instead, we followed the suggestion of Staley et al., and used fluorescent-labeled skin markers.

Standard techniques and procedures that presented no unusual difficulties need only be mentioned and referenced.

> We measured hair loss using the standard method of Kojak.

Quality

A central issue in nearly every study is whether the main outcome measurements were performed *blindly,* that is, without knowledge of the underlying research hypothesis. The need for blinding has been emphasized in clinical trials: It serves to prevent investigators from "improving" the outcome of a patient whom they know to be in the group receiving the active drug. But blinding is also important in many other types of clinical research. If, for example, you hypothesize that people who wear eyeglasses are more intelligent, and you measure intelligence by your opinion as to how well participants interpret proverbs, then you may erroneously bias your results. In lieu of blinding, sometimes measurements are made according to a standardized protocol, such as an IQ test. This prevents flexibility bias. (The same concerns about blinding should also apply to animal and bench research, although reviewers seldom seem concerned about blinding measurements in these studies.)

For many variables, especially those that measure "soft stuff" such as pain or quality of life, discuss the validity and reliability of any nonstandard measurement techniques that you used. *Validity* indicates whether what you measured has any meaning. Validity can be ascertained by comparison with a gold standard (someone else's way of measuring pain), by comparison with an "objective" measurement (use of pain medication), or by whether your measurement makes sense. *Reliability* indicates whether you would get the same result if you repeated the measurement; it is best ascertained by doing just that, at least with a sample.

ANALYSIS

The Analysis section of your paper poses two big problems. First, the completion of data analysis usually happens at the same time you are writing the results of the study. Indeed, sometimes the paper is mostly written while the analyses are just beginning. Thus, analysis tends to be the most "fluid" section of the manuscript. You can make changes in the analyses, and, therefore, in the Analysis section of the methods, with greater ease and at a later time than you can change who was in the study or how you measured the variables. Second, there is a strong temptation to list the statistical tests (or worse, the software program) that you used rather than describe the actual analysis plan in English.

> We use *t* tests, chi-squared tests, linear regression, and some other kind of fancy test whose name we cannot remember but that our statistician recommended as state of the art and swore that no one would understand anyway; we certainly did not.

Instead, describe how and why you analyzed your data. This includes discussing how you determined the effect size, which subjects were in which analyses, whether you transformed your data, how you evaluated the statistical significance of your results, and how you checked for alternative explanations. Tell the reader why you chose the analytic method you used.

> Because of differences in baseline characteristics in the two groups, all analyses were adjusted for age (in years), race (black, white, and others), sex, and socio-economic status (years of education) using logistic regression models.

Effect Size

Make sure you describe the key effect size clearly and that it corresponds to your research hypothesis (for a complete discussion of effect sizes, see Chapter 5). For example, if your research hypothesis was that drug A is better than drug B at reducing serum glucose levels in patients with diabetes, then your effect size is the mean difference in the changes in glucose levels in the two groups—a difference of the differences. If your research hypothesis is that final serum glucose levels are lower after treatment with drug A than with drug B, then your effect size is the mean difference in the final values in the two groups. If your research hypothesis is that the percentage reduction in serum glucose is greater with drug A than with drug B, your effect size is the mean difference in the percentage change between the two groups, and you will need to specify how you defined "percentage change."

Explain what you did to measure the effect sizes in clear terms. Begin with the main effect size, then move on to secondary outcome variables and more sophisticated techniques. Discuss the statistical tests you used to demonstrate that the effects were statistically significant.

> We compared the risk of myocardial infarction in those taking nonsteroidal agents and those taking aspirin, expressed as a risk difference and as a risk ratio; we assessed the statistical significance of these effects using the chi-squared test. Next, we used proportional hazards models to adjust for the effects of age, education, and body weight (as continuous variables); for the effects of smoking (ever, never, and past) as a categorical variable; and for the presence of current diabetes and previous myocardial infarction as dichotomous variables.

If you used the same statistical test to ascertain several effect sizes, you need not repeat the technique over and over.

Change:

> We compared mean weights using the *t* test. We compared mean blood pressure using the *t* test. Length of stay was compared using the rank-sum test. We compared total hospital costs with rank-sum tests.

To:

> We compared mean differences using the *t* test, or the rank-sum test when data were skewed (i.e., length of stay and total hospital costs).

Certain statistical methods, such as analysis of variance (ANOVA) and correlation, do not correspond to easily understandable effect sizes. This becomes a problem when the use of such a statistical technique has become standard in the field (as ANOVA is in psychology and physiology). You may, for example, have compared mean low-density lipoprotein (LDL) cholesterol levels in three groups fed different diets (high, medium, and low fiber). Any biostatistician worth her salt will tell you that you cannot compare the mean LDL cholesterol levels in each of the possible pairs of groups (high vs. medium fiber, high vs. low fiber, and medium vs. low fiber) without first showing that there is an overall difference among the three groups. In other words, do an ANOVA. But that does not let you off the hook of having to describe how you *measured* the effect sizes.

> We measured mean LDL cholesterol levels after 6 months on the different diets; the changes from baseline were compared.

Who Was Analyzed?

You must describe whether all the subjects were included in every analysis, or whether certain subjects were excluded, and, if so, when. Ideally, you will have a similar number of subjects for each of your analyses, but sometimes that is not the case. Suppose, for example, you started the study with 300 patients and have base-line data on 250 of them. After 2 years of follow-up, data are available only on 150 of those subjects. The reader needs to be made aware of these differences, and, if it matters, be told how the 50 subjects with missing data as well as the 100 subjects without follow-up differed from the 150 with complete data.

Sometimes, the number of subjects in the study is much larger than the number in the actual analyses. This is especially true if multivariable modeling techniques are used because any subject with missing data for any of the variables in the model will be excluded (unless you use special techniques to impute the values of the missing data). This may lead you to make false conclusions based on the (much) smaller sample size, especially because subjects with complete data are often not representative of the entire group. Always include the number of subjects included in multivariate models.

Variable Transformation

The way you measured a variable and the way you treat it in the analyses may not be the same. For example, you may have measured education in several cat-egories (grade school, some high school, high school, some college, college, etc.) but treated education as a dichotomous variable (some college or greater vs. high school or less) in the analyses. If the variable matters a great deal (as it would if your research hypothesis concerned the effects of education on the incidence of depression), then you should describe in complete detail how the variable was measured, and explain how it was treated. However, be consistent in all sections of the manuscript. If you dichotomized a variable (age <65 years, ≥65 years) in your data analysis, provide the percentage of subjects in each of those two groups in the results, rather than merely providing the mean age, thereby leaving the reader to guess how many subjects were aged 65 years or older.

If you averaged a measurement made on a few occasions, say so. If you elimi-nated certain measurements because they did not make sense, that should also be made clear.

Some variables (such as length of hospital stay) have a very asymmetric distribu-tion that may violate the assumptions that underlie a particular statistical test. Some-times, it is worthwhile to transform this sort of variable (e.g., by taking its logarithm). Another type of transformation involves having a hierarchical classification scheme. Say, for instance, that you are studying risk factors for epithelial cancer. If someone had a skin cancer, an adenomatous colon polyp, and a gastric cancer, how did you classify her? If someone used to be a pipe smoker, then a cigar smoker, but was a cigarette smoker during your study, how was he classified?

Adjustment

Were all your analyses adjusted for age or other factors? If so, then stating that once in the Methods section is much more efficient than constantly repeating "in an age-adjusted analysis" in the Results section.

How did you determine what to adjust for? Did you choose important adjust-ment variables on the basis of a review of the literature? Did you make your choices on the basis of common sense or some sort of statistical criteria?

Elaborate statistical models, such as linear regression, logistic regression, and Cox proportional hazards models, have criteria that are concerned with issues such as how you decided to include or exclude a variable and what you did with missing data. These may matter a great deal and should be mentioned. These models also make assumptions about the underlying structure of the data. Be sure to mention whether you tested the validity of those assumptions. If you are not familiar with those assumptions, see the appendix to Chapter 5 (Results) for more details; more important, obtain statistical help.

Change:

We used multivariable logistic regression to analyze our data.

To:

To adjust for the effects of potential confounders, we used logistic regression models. We verified that the associations between continuous predictors and the outcomes were linear in the log odds by examining odds by quintile of the predictors, and by including quadratic terms in the models.

If you do not understand the statistical methods that were used in your study well enough to explain them to the reader, then you should not have used them. This does not mean that you must understand the theory underlying the procedures. If you are working with a statistician, you do not have to know the assumptions that underlie the particular tests. That is the statistician's job. But you have to know enough to be able to write about the rationale for using the tests or at least to edit what your statistical colleagues have written.

Power

If you did a power calculation before your study, the Analysis section is the place to mention it. However, at the end of a study, the confidence intervals around the main results matter much more than the power calculations you did before you started the study. Why? Because power calculations were based on what you *thought* might happen in the study; confidence intervals are based on what actually did happen. Unfortunately, many—and perhaps even most—journal editors and reviewers do not understand this point. Thus even if you have provided confidence intervals, they will often insist that you also provide information about the estimated power.

All sentences that include the word *power* also need to include the sample size, the effect size and its variability, and the alpha level (if those terms do not make sense, read Chapters 5 and 6 in *Designing Clinical Research*[1]). A statement such as "We had 90% power to show a difference" is meaningless. This is not an exaggeration. You need a statement that includes all the relevant terms.

With 245 subjects in each group, we had 90% power to detect a two fold difference in the risk of wrist fracture between the two groups, assuming a risk of 5% in the control group, at an alpha (two-sided) of 0.05.

We estimated that we would require a total of 128 subjects evenly divided into the two groups to detect whether the intervention was associated with a 10 mg/dL difference in final blood glucose levels between the groups, assuming a standard deviation of 20 mg/dL for blood glucose levels, at a power of 80% and a two-sided alpha of 0.05 and no loss to follow-up.

If you are at your wit's end about how to write such a sentence, seek help from a biostatistician (preferably before doing the study!).

You should also describe how you determined whether a result was statistically significant.

We considered P values <0.05 as statistically significant; all tests were two-sided.

Because of the large number of hypotheses, we used a criterion of <0.01 for determining statistical significance.

We estimated 95% confidence intervals for the main results.

Conclude by mentioning, if appropriate, the statistical software packages you used. Provide references for any special analytic techniques.

SPECIAL SITUATIONS

Randomized Controlled Trials

Usually, if you are responsible for presenting the results of a randomized trial, you have enough help from senior investigators and biostatisticians that you will not have to face the problem of writing the manuscript by yourself. Indeed, you are likely to have the opposite problem of too many coauthors meddling with your work. However, there may be times when you have done a small clinical trial without a great deal of external support or without any experienced colleagues and need guidance on how to prepare your results for publication. There are now standard criteria, assembled by a group of investigators and journal editors, for reporting the results of randomized trials; see the website at www.consort-statement.org. Many journals require that you provide the answers to all of the questions in the Consort documents.

Several points warrant special attention. *First,* was everyone who was enrolled in the study assigned to one of the treatment groups? *Second,* how were patients assigned to the different treatment groups (i.e., was that process truly random)? *Third,* what did the intervention and control consist of? *Fourth,* were the outcomes ascertained and validated in the same way in the different groups, preferably without knowledge of which group the patients had been assigned to? *Fifth,* were follow-up data available on all the participants? *Sixth,* did the investigators define the main outcome of the trial in advance, and was that prespecified outcome used in determining whether the treatment was effective? *Finally,* was the outcome compared among all patients who were enrolled in the study?

The last requirement—sometimes called the *once randomized, always analyzed* rule—can seem problematic. Consider, for example, a placebo-controlled study of a new treatment for septic shock. Enrollment criteria are developed (hypotension, no hemorrhage or trauma, no evidence of heart failure, lactate level >4 mmol/L, etc.), and patients are enrolled and randomly assigned to either the treatment or the control group. Further diagnostic tests, such as blood cultures, are available only 2 or 3 days later; the investigators believe that enrolling patients at that time will be too late. Thus, it turns out that half of the patients (about equally divided between the treatment and control groups) did not really have septic shock. Which groups should be compared: the original treatment and control groups, or just those that turned out to have positive blood cultures?

A similar problem arises when patients cross over from one randomly assigned treatment (e.g., surgical therapy for breast cancer) to another treatment (radiation). Which groups should be compared: those originally assigned to each of the treatments or those that ended up with the treatment?

Two points decide the question in favor of the "once randomized, always analyzed" rule. First, only the original groups were assigned randomly. Therefore, only the original group assignments maintain the chief advantage of the randomization process, which is to ensure the comparability of the two groups. As soon as subjects are withdrawn from the study, for whatever reason, one cannot be sure that the remaining groups are comparable. Second, it is essential to keep in mind the clinical question. A clinician considering a new therapy for sepsis would not have the luxury of waiting 2 to 3 days for the blood culture results; he or she would need to decide on the basis of incomplete information. Thus, your study must convince the clinician that the therapy is beneficial among patients who *might* have sepsis.

Studies of a Diagnostic (or Prognostic) Test

The characteristics of the sample matter a great deal in studies of diagnostic and prognostic tests. Were the patients compared with healthy controls or with subjects with similar presentation in whom the diagnosis was also being realistically considered? It is less clinically relevant to evaluate a diagnostic test that can distinguish patients with pancreatitis from healthy controls; it will be better to show that the test works in separating patients with pancreatitis from those with other causes of abdominal pain. Did the subjects with the disease tend to have advanced cases (as often happens at referral centers, where much clinical research is performed), or was their disease in its early stages?

You should also discuss the issue of blinding. Did the results of the diagnostic test influence the ultimate diagnosis, or did the diagnosis influence how the diagnostic test was interpreted? Although it may seem obvious to you, as the author, that the laboratory technician who determined the serum oxalate level could not have known whether a patient had kidney stones, this will not be apparent to reviewers and readers unless you specifically say so.

Synthetic Studies

The methods used in synthetic studies (decision analysis, cost-effectiveness analysis, and meta-analysis) can be difficult to describe. It is tempting to provide a broad overview ("We based estimates of complication rates from the literature") rather than cite specific sources for each item in your analysis. Although you may be eventually asked by the journal editor to provide a summary to conserve space, it is generally a mistake to do so at the manuscript review stage. There are enough experts in the different techniques who are familiar with the nitty-gritty of the methods involved that you can be reasonably sure that your manuscript will be carefully evaluated for "methodologic rigor." It is also likely that another reviewer who is familiar with the clinical problem will be asked to review your manuscript. You must satisfy both types of reviewers.

Someone who reads your Methods section should be able to re-create your study. Indeed, as most synthetic studies are based on previously published or otherwise available results, the reader should also be able to re-create your exact results. This puts you at a disadvantage relative to someone doing primary research. Reviewers may select the most important results of your study, the strangest results, or the ones that interest them most and try to duplicate them. If the reviewers are unsuccessful, they will inevitably question your entire analysis. Ensure that this does not happen by spelling out the exact methods and data sources you used.

MISCELLANEOUS POINTS

What Is a Result, and What Is a Method?

Suppose you are doing a survey of attitudes about returning mailed surveys. You had a list of 1,000 potential subjects and were able to find addresses or phone numbers for 850 of them, of which 650 appeared to be valid. Of those who reviewed the survey, 500 responded in some form; 400 filled out the questionnaire completely. Does this information belong in the Results section or in the Methods section? It depends on which way is easier for the reader to follow. If you can describe your methodology without using the numbers, and if the numbers can be understood when presented in the results, then do so. But sometimes it is easier to tell the reader what you did ("Of the 200 subjects without valid addresses or phone numbers, we were able to contact a relative or close friend in 125 cases, of which...") in the Methods section.

The Not-Quite-Perfect Study

What if there is a discrepancy between what you actually did and how you wish you had done the study, or how you want to describe your methods? For example, you may have intended to study every patient with temporal arteritis seen at your hospital in the past 2 years. However, some charts were missing, and others were incomplete. When you discover that some of the patients diagnosed with temporal arteritis had other conditions, you suddenly realize that there must have been other patients with temporal arteritis who went undiagnosed. The laboratory may have changed how it measured the erythrocyte sedimentation rate in the middle of the study period.

Clinical research is never perfect, so there is no need to pretend otherwise. Avoid being less than honest. Acknowledge the little errors. Do not gloss over imperfections in your methods. If you used a less-than-ideal method of measurement ("Self-reported weight was recorded") or did not find every potential subject in the same way ("Some subjects were recruited through postcard mailings; others were identified from lists of clinic patients"), then say so. Remember that reviewers are almost always researchers, and they understand that the world of research is messy. They also value honesty.

Sometimes, no one can remember where the subjects came from, or exactly how a particular measurement was made. Not uncommonly, a neophyte investigator inherits data that were collected several years before, but never analyzed ("Here's a good project for you; go write it up"). If you cannot track down the research assistant or fellow who originally worked on the project (hint: ask around among the administrative and technical personnel, who usually know more about where people are than the principal investigator does), what can you do? Confess: "These data were collected during 2005 to 2007, and the exact methods used to assess pulmonary function are not known." Confession can prevent the horribly embarrassing situation of having someone write a letter to the editor about your data: "Contrary to Dr. Barnum's statement that participants were volunteer medical school faculty, the subjects in this study were actually clowns recruited from a visiting circus."

✔ CHECKLIST FOR

METHODS

1. Could another scientist reproduce your study on the basis of the details you provided?

2. Did you mention the design of the study?

3. Are the setting, source and number of subjects, and inclusion and exclusion criteria for subjects clear?

4. Are the measurements described in a logical order with the appropriate level of detail? Are quality issues addressed?

5. Did you state how you measured the effect size and how you determined whether it was statistically significant?

6. Did you describe any data transformations or sophisticated analytic techniques and explain why you used them?

7. Do any special features need to be mentioned?

8. Have you followed the Consort guideline (www.consort-statement.org) if you are reporting the results of a randomized trial?

Reference

1. Hulley SB, Cummings SR, Browner WS, et al., eds. *Designing Clinical Research: An Epidemiologic Approach*. 3rd ed. Philadelphia, PA: Lippincott Williams & Wilkins; 2007.

5 Results

Unless you introduce a brilliant new scientific technique in the Methods section or propose an extraordinarily innovative theory in your discussion, the Results section of your study will constitute the major scientific contribution of your manuscript. So it is worth spending time to get this section of the manuscript as close to perfect as you can. Moreover, most investigators have more to learn about presenting results than about any other part of the manuscript.

The biggest mistake authors make in the Results section involves confusing data with information. Anything you can measure can become data, but only those data that have meaning can become information. The distinction is critical. Information is always useful; data may or may not be. You are not obligated to present every possible result from your study, only those that are relevant. Including too many pieces of data just obscures the important stuff. Readers do not need to be told the mean, median, standard deviation (SD), standard error, confidence interval, and range of every measurement you made. You may have measured the sphingomyelin levels in cerebrospinal fluid every 15 minutes for 24 hours, but unless these measurements are meaningful, they should not be included in the results.

Be prepared to analyze, and perhaps even collect, more data as you write. In your eagerness to finish a manuscript, this may not seem very appealing. You may have little interest in doing more analyses or making more measurements. But research is an iterative process. As you write the Results section, you may realize that you have not actually finished your study. If you just cannot face the possibility of collecting or analyzing more data, imagine adding a paragraph like the one below to the cover letter describing your study to a journal editor:

> Please consider this manuscript for publication in the *Journal of Hasty Investigators,* even though we did not have information on caffeine consumption, which we forgot to record in our chart abstraction sheets. Although it may appear essential to have data on caffeine use in a study about sleep, we simply did not have the energy to review the medical records. We thought it was more important to submit an incomplete manuscript, and hope that you and the reviewers will agree.

Perhaps the commonest mistake that young investigators (and some senior ones, too) make is writing a manuscript around a significant P value: "We found no relation between beverage consumption and inflammatory bowel disease, except that people who drank between one and three pints of bottled water daily were 34% more likely to have ulcerative colitis than expected ($P < 0.03$)." Unless you had prespecified that specific hypothesis before you did your analyses (presumably on the basis of a prior study that had a similarly weird result), this kind of oddball result is almost certainly due to chance. Resist the temptation of believing otherwise.

This fundamental point is so important that it needs repeating: Do not write a manuscript (or abstract) around a significant P value. Write your manuscript around the main findings of your study—whether they are statistically significant or not.

Similarly, do not rely on statistical jargon to describe the results: "We found a significant interaction among the variables ($F_{3,111}$ = 5.1, P = 0.002)." Say what it is that you found: "We found that the effects of education on income varied by race, such that higher education had a greater effect in Hispanic Americans than in other ethnic and racial groups (P = 0.002)."

To clarify the proper role of statistics in your study, it may be useful to use a theatrical analogy. If the title of your play (study) is *My Research Question* (what you were studying), then its star is the *effect size* (what you found), with supporting roles for the effect size's *confidence interval* (the precision of what you found) and, if needed, *adjusted analyses* (the exploration of alternative explanations), with a cameo appearance by the P value (which, although its career is fading slowly, insisted on being included). Do not let a P value—or an F statistic or a χ^2 test—steal the show. The effect size must take center stage.

That said, this chapter provides an overview of statistics that is meant to help you understand the purpose of statistical tests in clinical research by providing a context for them. It is not intended as a substitute for either learning about statistics yourself or getting the help of statistically savvy colleagues.

Most people do not think of means, risks, or odds ratios—the material covered in the first part of this chapter—when they hear the word *statistics,* even though all these terms are, in fact, statistics. To keep things simple, these sorts of measures will be referred to as estimates or point estimates. The term *statistics* will be reserved for things such as P values, confidence intervals, and t tests. Before talking about how to organize a Results section, let us cover the different kinds of results that will appear in it.

DESCRIPTIVE AND ANALYTIC RESULTS

More likely than not, your manuscript will have two basic types of results: *descriptive* and *analytic*. Each type requires its own type of statistics—more on that later. Descriptive results involve only one variable, either a predictor or an outcome. The following are examples of descriptive results:

> We enrolled 112 men with stomach cancer, 35% (n = 31) of whom were smokers.

> The mean (±SD) age of our subjects was 67 ± 12 years.

> During the first month of follow-up, 460 (23%) of the patients with heart failure were readmitted to the hospital.

It is usually a good idea to include the actual numbers and the percentages as double check. (Note, for example, that 35% of 112 is actually 39, not 31! So at least one of the three numbers—112, 35%, or 31—must be wrong.)

Descriptive results can include more than one variable, so long as you do not compare them, as in the example below:

> We enrolled 78 men and 34 women.

Of the 198 subjects, 40 (20%) smoked, 16 (8%) had diabetes, and 9 (5%) had previous myocardial infarction.

Mean (±SD) systolic blood pressure was 142 ± 12 mm Hg in men and 138 ± 9 mm Hg in women.

Sometimes, a descriptive result in your sample is a point estimate of the actual value in the broader population from which your sample was drawn. The "23%" who were readmitted might be an estimate of the proportion of all patients with heart failure who are readmitted, if you surveyed a random sample of admitted patients in the United States. On the other hand, it might not be, if, for example, you drew your sample from communities with poor follow-up systems.

Analytic results, by contrast, involve the comparison of two or more variables or groups. Certain words suggest that your results are analytic:

Compared with, in contrast, more, greater, bigger, higher, less, fewer, lower, similar to, relative risk, odds ratio, twice as likely as, related to, associated with, correlated with.

Do not be fooled. The following simple "descriptions" of what happened are actually analytic results.

We found that boys were more likely than girls to have been called into the principal's office.

Of our 93 subjects, fewer had diabetes than hypertension.

Mean glucose level was 10 mg/dL greater in patients with asthma than in controls.

Analytic results and their statistics—such as confidence intervals and *P* values—are discussed later in the chapter.

Types of Descriptive Data

Descriptive data come in three basic varieties: *dichotomous, categorical,* and *continuous.*

Dichotomous, or binary, data can have only one of two values, such as yes or no; currently drinks or does not drink alcohol; dead or alive. Dichotomous data happen to, or are an attribute of, each subject. Examples of dichotomous variables include death, myocardial infarction, having a history of osteoarthritis, and visiting a dentist at least once in the previous year.

Categorical data can have a limited number of mutually exclusive possibilities, such as "poor, fair, good, or excellent," or "internist, surgeon, or pediatrician." *Mutually exclusive* means that someone cannot fill two possibilities simultaneously—cannot, for example, be classified as both an internist and a surgeon (at least for the purposes of your study!). There are two types of categorical data: *ordinal data,* which have a logical order, such as annual income under $10,000, $10,000 to $19,999, $20,000 to $39,999, or $40,000 and over; and *nominal data,* which do not have a logical sequence, for example, the blood groups O, A, B, and AB. (Therefore, type of physician would be nominal, whereas mean physician income by $50,000 per year increments would be ordinal.) If you do have overlapping categories (such as hobbies—some people have several), then you need another category, such as "more than one."

Alternatively, you can list the primary hobby, perhaps by time spent in an average week.

Continuous data, such as body weight or serum potassium level, can theoretically have an infinite number of values. Any limitation placed on the possibilities is simply one of precision. For example, we do not distinguish between a potassium level of 4.12 mEq/L and one of 4.13 mEq/L, but we could. In practice, data that can have 6 (some say 10) or more ordered values are often regarded as continuous.

Any variable can be made dichotomous by introducing a cut point or by lumping categories together. You may have measured height to the nearest millimeter, but the variable can be dichotomized into tall (≥190 cm) or not tall (<190 cm).

Describing Dichotomous and Categorical Variables

Describing dichotomous and categorical data is easy. Simply provide the number or the percentage, and sometimes both, of the subjects with each characteristic:

> Of the 158 subjects, 12 (8%) had undergone previous oral surgery.

> About half (48% [$n = 101$]) of the 211 subjects were medical students; the rest were either pharmacy students (22% [$n = 46$]), graduate students (15% [$n = 32$]), laboratory employees (9% [$n = 19$]), or others (6% [$n = 13$]).

> The 5-year risk of pulmonary involvement was 12% (13 of 111) among women with rheumatoid arthritis, and 23% (14 of 62) among those with lupus erythematosus.

> The sensitivity of the anti-Jenner antibody for the diagnosis of Lyme disease was 50% (17 of 34).

Provide the numerator each time and the denominator (at least once); doing so helps the reader determine the precision of that percentage: 4 of 10 and 394 of 986 are both 40%, but the second estimate is more precise. Indicate precision by using the appropriate number of digits when describing your results. For example, 4 of 22 is 18%, not 18.18%. (One could argue that 4/22 is better approximated as 20%, except that the apparent math error would be distracting.) Better yet, just say 4 of 22. Some journals do not allow the use of percentages if the denominator is small, say, <50.

With a dichotomous variable, if you know what proportion of subjects has one of the values, you also know the proportion that has the other value. For example, if 10% of the subjects were men, then 90% must have been women. You should not present the proportion of men and the proportion of women; choose one from each dichotomous pair.

Change:

> Of the 196 subjects, 86 (44%) were alive and 110 (56%) were dead at the end of the study.

To:

> After 3 years, 44% (86 of 196) of the subjects were still alive.

Change:

> We enrolled 93 subjects, 30% of whom had diabetes and 70% of whom did not.

To:

We enrolled 93 subjects, of whom 30% (28) had diabetes.

For categorical variables, you should provide the proportions for each group because the reader will not necessarily know what the remaining category describes.

Change:

We found that 12% of the subjects had poor health, 23% had fair health, and 41% had good health.

To:

Of the 331 subjects, 12% (*n* = 40) reported poor health, 23% (*n* = 76) fair health, 41% (*n* = 136) good health, and 24% (*n* = 79) excellent health.

Sometimes you may have a composite dichotomous variable. Suppose, for example, you are studying whether cardiovascular events are more common in persons with high *Chlamydia trachomatis* titers. *Cardiovascular events* is a composite variable, consisting of the occurrence of any of the following: stroke, myocardial infarction, heart failure, or cardiovascular death. A subject who had two strokes and a myocardial infarction, and then later dies suddenly is counted as having only one dichotomous outcome (cardiovascular event = yes), not four.

Risks, rates, and *odds* are estimates of the frequency of a dichotomous outcome in a group of subjects who have been followed for a specific period. These three measures are closely related. They share the same numerator, which is the number of subjects who have the dichotomous outcome. Implicit in these three measures is the concept of being *at risk,* which means that the subject did not already have the outcome of interest at the beginning of the study. In a prospective study of the predictors of diabetes, a woman who had diabetes at baseline would not be *at risk* because she already had the outcome of interest. (On the other hand, there are episodic diseases such as gout or heart failure requiring admission to a hospital, in which the outcome you are interested in may be the "incident" occurrence of a new episode, even if it occurs in someone who already has the disease.)

Consider, for example, a study of 5,000 people who were followed for 2 years to see who developed lung cancer and among whom 80 new cases occurred. Risk, odds, and rate are estimated as follows.

Measurement	Formula	Example
Risk	$\dfrac{N \text{ who develop the outcome}}{N \text{ at risk}}$	$\dfrac{80}{5{,}000} = 0.016$
Odds	$\dfrac{N \text{ who develop the outcome}}{N \text{ who do not develop the outcome}}$	$\dfrac{80}{4{,}920} = 0.0163$
Rate	$\dfrac{N \text{ who develop the outcome}}{\text{Person-time at risk}}$	$\dfrac{80}{9{,}960 \text{ person-years}}$ $= 0.008 \text{ per person-year}$

Person-time is defined as the total amount of follow-up for the sample; each subject contributes to that total so long as that subject is alive, remains in the study, and has not yet had the outcome.

Of the three measures, risk is the easiest to understand, perhaps because of its everyday familiarity. Although it may not be intuitively obvious why you would ever want to use odds, they are essential in two situations: when you have done a case–control study and when you use logistic regression. Rate has certain biologically attractive characteristics. After all, the amount of follow-up time should certainly matter when describing the frequency of a disease or outcome. However, rate requires the most epidemiologic knowledge to understand and estimate.

If an outcome occurs in <10% of the sample, then risk and odds are approximately the same. For example, a 5-year risk of 8 per 100 persons (0.08) equals an odds of 0.09. And when the outcome is rare, risk is also similar to the rate multiplied by the average amount of follow-up time. But when outcome is common, the measures can be very different. For example, a risk of 0.9 corresponds to an odds of 9.

When reporting, risk, rate, or odds do not inflate the denominator beyond the sample size. Suppose you tracked 60 women with osteoporosis for an average of 2 years during which 8 women suffered vertebral fractures. Do not claim that the vertebral fracture rate was 667 per 10,000 person-years: your study had only about 120 person-years of follow-up. Say that the fracture rate was about 7 per 100 person-years; at least the denominator is in the same ballpark as your sample.

Sometimes, such as in a cross-sectional study, the concepts of *at risk* or *who develop* do not apply. Instead, describe the frequency of a dichotomous variable as its *prevalence:*

$$\text{Prevalence} = \frac{\text{Number with a characteristic}}{\text{Total number of subjects}}$$

For example, the prevalence of myopia among medical students might be 25% (38 per 150).

Describing Continuous Variables

When describing a continuous variable, provide the reader with the *sort-of-average* value of the variable and a sense of how much *spread,* or variation, there was in that variable in your sample. I've used the terms "sort of average" and "spread," rather than technically correct terms, to make a point: It matters which technical term you should use. If the values of a continuous variable are normally distributed (or bell shaped, or close to symmetrical around the sort of average), then they should be described by the mean, which is the average value, and the SD, which measures the spread. If the values are skewed—in other words, almost everything else—they are often better described by the median and the interquartile range (the 25th and 75th percentiles).

The sort of average and spread of a variable provide the reader with information about the population from which your sample was chosen and to which your results may apply. This explains why you should use the median for skewed data: When describing the sort-of-average income in a sample, one or two rich persons can make the mean income ridiculously high. In that situation, the median provides a better sense of the sort-of-average value. This also explains why SDs are preferable to standard errors. The SD indicates the spread of the variable in the sample, thereby estimating the spread in that variable in the population from which the sample was drawn. It does not depend on the size of the sample. The standard error of the mean, conversely, does depend on the sample size. It equals the SD divided by the square root of the sample size, and it is an estimate of how precisely the mean in the sample has been measured. If you have a big enough sample, you will have a very small standard error. But the standard error does not tell the reader anything about the spread of the variable.

Many authors prefer to use standard errors because they are always smaller, and sometimes much smaller, than SD. If it matters how precisely you estimated a mean value of a descriptive result—and it seldom does—then provide the 95% confidence interval for the mean (which equals the mean plus or minus about twice the standard error).

Continuous data should be described with the same level of precision that was used to make the measurement. This is one of the commonest errors that authors make.

Change:

Systolic blood pressure (mean ± SD) was 122.85 ± 12.44 mm Hg.

Mean (±SD) weight in men was 70.285 ± 4.942 kg.

To:

Systolic blood pressure (mean ± SD) was 123 ± 12 mm Hg.

Mean (± SD) weight in men was 70.3 ± 4.9 kg.

The same principle holds for self-reported values. If you asked subjects the number of packs of cigarettes they smoked per day to the nearest half-pack, do not report that they smoked a mean of 27.6 cigarettes per day.

Use the appropriate units for the journal to which you plan to send your manuscript. If the journal requires that you use Système International (SI) units or report the conversion factor, then do so. But beware the problem of introducing excessive precision through multiplication or division. As an example, consider converting cholesterol values from SI units to mg per dL; the conversion factor is mg per dL = 38.7 × mmol/L. If the mean cholesterol was 6.1 mmol/L in your sample, this would be equivalent to 6.1 × 38.7 = 236.07 mg/dL. But because serum cholesterol in SI units is measured to the nearest 0.1 mmol/L (which is about 4 mg/dL), it would be better to report the mean value as 236 mg/dL.

Try not to be tricked into thinking that risk is a continuous variable. Risk is a way to report how frequently a dichotomous outcome occurred; it is not an outcome variable. The same holds true for rates and odds.

Analytic Results

Analytic results involve comparisons, usually between two groups (e.g., men are heavier than women; lung cancer is more common in smokers than nonsmokers). First you must decide who should be compared. In a randomized trial, the primary analysis follows the principle known as *intention-to-treat,* also called *once randomized, always analyzed.* The primary comparison is between the subjects who were initially assigned to the different groups. This holds true whether they received the designated intervention or completed the study, for the reasons discussed in Chapter 4 (Special Situations: Randomized Controlled Trials). Other types of studies should usually strive to emulate this principle by comparing groups that are as similar as possible, except for the particular variable of interest.

Consider a study of whether exposure to aerosols is a risk factor for lung cancer. The investigators are not interested in smoking, as this is already known to be an important risk factor. The effects of smoking can be dealt with in the design phase of the study, by matching cases of lung cancer and controls for smoking status; a case who smoked would be matched with a control who smoked, and vice versa. Another design phase strategy would involve choosing only nonsmoking cases and controls. Comparing "like with like" can also be accomplished in the analysis phase of the study, by doing separate comparisons of the association between aerosol use and lung cancer in smokers and nonsmokers. A common analysis-phase strategy involves determining the effect of aerosol use on lung cancer after adjusting for differences in smoking with multivariable models. These are discussed in more detail later in the chapter.

A second analytical principle involves making comparisons *between* groups, rather than *within* a group. This is especially important for randomized trials that evaluate the effect of a therapy on a continuous outcome. For example, consider a placebo-controlled study of the effects of a new drug on weight loss. The appropriate analysis involves comparing the difference in change in weight between the placebo group and the treatment group. It would be inappropriate to compare the weights at the beginning and the end of the study in the treatment group and then state that subjects treated with the drug lost weight (maybe the same thing happened in the placebo group!).

Finally, it is essential to compare independent sampling units. For example, consider a study of whether acromegaly affects finger size. You should not test this hypothesis by comparing the mean circumference of 10 fingers in a single patient with acromegaly with the mean circumference of 10 fingers in a single control. The problem, of course, is that the circumference of any one finger in an individual is correlated with that of the other fingers. Similarly, in a study of angioedema, five episodes in a single patient should not be counted as five separate sampling units.

What Should Be Compared?

The *effect size* measures the magnitude of the difference between the two groups. Concentrating on the effect size will remind you to avoid writing a Results section around a significant P value. Remember, the effect size is the star; the P value is not. The best way to measure the effect size may not be obvious. Consider a study (Table 5.1) comparing interns with residents on the day after being on call.

TABLE 5.1	Characteristics of Interns and Residents the Day after Being on Call	
Characteristics	**Interns (_n_ = 40)**	**Residents (_n_ = 20)**
Alert in rounds	40%	60%
Mood		
Happy	20%	40%
Neutral	30%	30%
Sad	50%	30%
Sleep, mean hours per night	4.2	6.8

Even the simplest of the characteristics—the proportion who are alert—can be compared in a few ways. You can say that residents are 1.5 times as likely to be alert (60%/40% = 1.5), or 20% more likely (60% – 40%). You can also say that interns are 0.67 times as likely to be alert, or 20% less likely. Worse still, you could also say that residents are 50% more likely to be alert, because (60% – 40%)/40% = 50%, or that interns are 33% less likely to be alert, since (60% – 40%)/60% = 33%.

If you are not yet thoroughly confused by how arbitrary effect sizes can be, imagine what can happen with a categorical variable such as mood, or a continuous variable such as hours of sleep, or if a third group is added. And what if you want to do some sort of multivariable analysis?

Given the potential for confusion, it becomes all too easy to rely on elaborate statistical models or lists of P values when presenting analytic results. A better strategy is to determine the most important effect sizes in your study and design your presentation around them.

Effect Sizes: A Systematic Approach

A single study can have several, and sometimes several hundred, effect sizes. These might include comparison of different outcomes, the same outcome at different times, or the results in different subgroups. No manuscript can possibly include all of these effect sizes. Instead, as you prepare to write the Results section, list the 5 or 10 most essential analytic results in your study. Do not despair if you have fewer: Brevity is a virtue. This first step of listing the key results is crucial. You are guaranteed to have a difficult, if not impossible, time writing the Results section if you ignore this advice because you will find your Results section—and your manuscript—wandering about aimlessly.

Here is an example of some possible key results of a placebo-controlled randomized trial of the effects of a new antigout drug:

1. Subjects treated with a new antigout drug did better than those treated with placebo.
2. The higher the baseline uric acid level, the greater the likelihood of gout.
3. Gout was more common in the first few months of the study and less common in the last few months of the study.
4. In the treatment group, the amount of urate lowering was related to the likelihood of developing gout.
5. Urate levels were inversely associated with renal function.

The second step is to decide which is the predictor variable and which the outcome variable for each of your key results. Keep in mind that the predictor variable can simply be "group assignment" (in this situation, treatment or control). Decide whether the predictor and outcome variables are dichotomous, categorical, or continuous. Each type has its own effect sizes.

Sometimes, this process is not as obvious as it appears. In reporting the results of the study of the antigout drug, does the main effect size compare the incidence of gouty episodes in the treatment and control groups, the serum urate levels in the two groups, the changes in serum urate levels, or the incidence of side effects in the two groups? Perhaps all four are important.

1. *Subjects treated with a new antigout drug did better than those treated with a placebo* =
   a. Dichotomous predictor (drug vs. placebo) and dichotomous outcome (occurrence of one or more symptomatic episodes of gout vs. no gout during follow-up)
   b. Dichotomous predictor (drug vs. placebo) and categorical outcome (felt better, the same, worse during follow-up)
   c. Dichotomous predictor (drug vs. placebo) and continuous outcome (serum urate level after 1 year)
   d. Dichotomous predictor (drug vs. placebo) and continuous outcome (change in serum urate level from baseline to 1 year)
   e. Dichotomous predictor (drug vs. placebo) and dichotomous outcome (side effects vs. none during follow-up)

2. *The higher the baseline uric acid level, the greater the likelihood of gout* = Continuous predictor (baseline urate level) and dichotomous outcome (gout vs. no gout during follow-up)

3. *Gout was more common in the first few months and less common in the last few months* = Categorical predictor (first 4 months vs. next 4 months vs. final 4 months) and dichotomous outcome (gout vs. no gout during each period)

4. *In the treatment group, the amount of urate lowering was related to the likelihood of developing gout* = Continuous predictor (change in urate level) and dichotomous outcome (gout vs. no gout during follow-up)

5. *Urate levels were inversely associated with renal function* = Continuous predictor (estimated creatinine clearance) and continuous outcome (baseline urate level)

The third step is to decide what sort of effect size to use, based on the type of predictor and outcome variables. Some examples of the most common effect sizes include risk ratios, odds ratios, mean differences, and correlations (Table 5.2).

The effect size measured in your study estimates the true effect size in the real world. That is, if you found that a new antigout drug reduced the risk of having an episode of gout by half in your study, then the best estimate is that the new drug will also reduce by half the risk of gout among all patients who are similar to those in your study. The effect size in the study is sometimes called the *point estimate,* and it is the single best estimate of the true effect size. Almost as important as determining the point estimate, however, is determining the *precision* of that estimate; there will be more on this fourth step later.

The list in Table 5.2 is not complete. For example, you may have used categorical variables. As a general rule, categorical outcome variables (e.g., better, the same, worse) should be avoided. If possible, the categories should be lumped together to make a dichotomous variable (better, same, or worse). The same lumping option is often the best choice for categorical predictor variables, although there are several other possibilities. One option is to select a base category to compare with the other categories. This makes the most sense, for example, for a clinical trial that has a placebo group, a low-dose drug and a higher-dose drug: In this situation, both treatment groups would logically be compared with the placebo group. It is also the only option if the categorical variable has no order. Consider, for example, a study of the effects of physician specialty (internal medicine, family practice, or gynecology) on cervical cancer screening. There is no logical order to these three groups, so you must arbitrarily pick a base category (e.g., internists) and compare the other groups with it.

TABLE 5.2 Effect Sizes

Predictor Variable	Outcome Variable	Effect Size	Formula with Example
Dichotomous	*Dichotomous*		
Male (vs. female)	Hypertension (SBP >160 or DBP >90)	Relative prevalence	$= \dfrac{\text{Proportion of men who are hypertensive}}{\text{Proportion of women who are hypertensive}}$
		Difference in prevalence	= Proportion of men who are hypertensive – Proportion of women who are hypertensive
Antistroke drug (vs. placebo)	Stroke in next 2 y	Risk ratio (relative risk)	$= \dfrac{\text{Risk of stroke in persons treated with drug}}{\text{Risk of stroke in persons treated with placebo}}$
		Risk difference	= Risk of stroke in persons treated with drug – Risk of stroke in persons treated with placebo
Use of saccharine (vs. nonuse)	Bladder cancer in next 20 y	Odds ratio[a] (cohort–study)	$= \dfrac{\text{Odds of cancer in users of saccharine}}{\text{Odds of cancer in non users}}$
Bladder cancer (vs. controls)	Use of saccharine in previous 20 y	Odds ratio[a] (case-control study)	$= \dfrac{\text{Odds of saccharine use in cases of cancer}}{\text{Odds of saccharine use in controls}}$
Vertebral fracture (vs. no vertebral fracture)	Hip fracture in next 5 y	Rate ratio (relative hazard)	$= \dfrac{\text{Hip fracture rate in those with vertebral fractures}}{\text{Hip fracture rate in those without vertebral fractures}}$
		Rate difference	= Rate of hip fracture in those with vertebral fractures – Rate of hip fracture in those without vertebral fractures

(Continued)

TABLE 5.2 Effect Sizes (Continued)

Predictor Variable	Outcome Variable	Effect Size	Formula with Example
Dichotomous	*Continuous*		
White (vs. non-white)	SBP	Mean difference	= Mean SBP in whites − Mean SBP in non-whites
		Mean percentage difference	$= \dfrac{\text{Mean SBP in whites} - \text{Mean SBP in non-whites}}{\text{Mean SBP in non whites}}$
New drug (vs. placebo)	Change in DBP	Mean difference in change	= Mean change in DBP in treatment group − Mean change in DBP in placebo group
Continuous	*Continuous*		
Creatinine clearance	1,25-Vitamin D level	Slope	= Change in 1,25-Vitamin D level per unit change in creatinine clearance
Serum lead level	IQ	Proportion of variance explained	= (Correlation between lead level and IQ)^2

[a]These two odds ratios—one from a cohort study and the other from a case–control study—are both estimates of the same odds ratio in the real world.

Another option, if the categories are ordered, is to compare each category with its nearest neighbor (low-dose with placebo, high-dose with low-dose). Finally, if there are enough categories (10 or more, and maybe even 6 or more), then treating the variable as if it were continuous may be the best choice.

You may have decided to use a more complicated effect size, such as the difference in the medians (as opposed to the means) in two groups if your data are skewed. For example, you may have done a study comparing length of hospital stay in two groups of patients. The basic principle of concentrating on the effect size remains the same; the only difference will be how you assess the precision of that estimate. This is discussed later in this chapter, under nonparametric tests. (In a study of diagnostic or prognostic tests, the effect size will be the characteristics of the test, such as sensitivity, specificity, and likelihood ratios. These are discussed in Chapter 12 of *Designing Clinical Research* (1).

In the next section of this chapter, effect sizes are discussed in more detail for each of the examples in Table 5.2.

Simple Effect Sizes for Dichotomous Predictor and Dichotomous Outcome Variables

Given all the choices, what is the preferred way to estimate the effect size for dichotomous predictor and outcome variables? The answer depends primarily on the design of the study. Is information available only about the prevalence of the outcome, as in a cross-sectional study? Was it a case–control study, which requires using odds ratios for the effect size? Were at-risk subjects followed for a specific period, as in a cohort study or a randomized trial? If so, this allows the use of risk, rate, or odds ratios, or risk or rate differences.

Risk ratios tell how *many times* more likely an event was to occur in one group than in another. There are several equivalent ways to express the same risk ratio. A risk ratio of 2.23 is the same as a 123% greater risk or a 2.23-fold greater risk. But you should avoid the phrase "123% greater risk" whenever possible; many readers will misunderstand you and those who do not have to add 100% to the 123% so they can arrive at the 2.23-fold greater risk.

With a dichotomous predictor variable (say, men vs. women), you can change a risk ratio of 3.0 into a risk ratio of 0.33 simply by changing the order of comparison, from men versus women to women versus men. But risk ratios (and odds ratios and rate ratios) that are <1.0 can be difficult to understand and often need to be explained. A risk ratio of 0.4 for head trauma means that the group with the predictor (e.g., wearing a bicycle helmet) had a risk that was 60% (1 − 0.4) lower than the other group's risk. In general, try to stick with risk ratios >1 and rephrase the results ("Those who did not wear bicycle helmets were 2.5 times more likely to have head injuries."). The exception is when reporting a randomized trial: Everyone is expecting risk ratios <1.0 for the comparison between the treatment and placebo groups because risk ratios <1 indicate that the treatment reduced the risk of the outcome (and, conversely, risk ratios >1 indicate that the treatment increased the risk of the outcome).

Risk differences tell how *much* more likely an outcome is to happen in one group than in another. They convey a sense of the absolute effect. A risk difference of 1% means that of 100 subjects, one less event occurred in one of the groups. A randomized trial with an event risk that was 1% lower in the intervention group than in the placebo group implies that 100 patients need to be treated to prevent one event. This statistic, known as the *number needed to treat* (NNT), is clinically quite useful.

$$NNT = \frac{1}{\text{Risk difference}}$$

For example, a risk difference of 3% corresponds to an NNT of 33 (= 1/0.03). NNTs are useful for the Discussion section of a manuscript because they provide a clinical context for the effect size.

You should be very cautious about using phrases such as "30% more likely" because the phrase can be interpreted as either 30% on an absolute scale as a risk difference (40% vs. 10%) or 30% on a relative scale (13% vs. 10%). If there is any chance that you might be misinterpreted, rephrase the sentence or provide the actual data. If you alternate between these different usages to avoid being repetitious, be sure you are not replacing dullness with confusion.

Rate ratios and rate differences are similar to risk ratios and risk differences; just substitute the word *rate* for *risk*. You can also estimate the NNT on the basis of rate differences.

$$NNT = \frac{1}{\text{Rate difference}}$$

For example, with a rate difference of 0.03 per person-year, the NNT would be 33 person-years. Indeed, by including an element of time, NNT based on rate differences gets around one of the main limitations of NNT calculated from risk differences. If you were told that among patients with mild-to-moderate hypertension, the NNT for antihypertensive treatment to prevent 1 stroke is 800, does that mean that 800 patients need to be treated for 1 year or for, say, 10 years? (The answer is per 1 year, approximately, which works out to about 80 patients treated for 10 years, a more reasonable way to describe the effects of treating a chronic risk factor like hypertension.)

Odds differences do not make sense and should not be used. When comparing odds, only the odds ratio is valid.

When an outcome is rare in the groups being compared, odds ratios, risk ratios, and rate ratios are similar. When the outcome is common (>10% in any group and especially if >30%), the three measures can be very different. For example, if the annual risk is 90% in one group and 80% in another, it corresponds to a risk ratio of 1.13 but to an odds ratio of 2.25 (= 9 ÷ 4). The rate ratio will be somewhere between the risk ratio and the odds ratio—in this example about 1.43. However, this does not mean that the risk ratio is intrinsically better than the other two measures; just that the terms are not interchangeable.

So how do you decide whether to present a risk difference or a risk ratio? Fortunately, this decision can be avoided because these two ways of expressing the effect size convey different types of information. If you provide the risk ratio in a table, then you should consider providing the risk difference in the text or vice versa.

More Complicated Ways to Express Effect Sizes for Dichotomous Predictor and Outcome Variables

More elaborate methods, such as the logistic regression model or the Cox proportional hazards model, allow you to adjust the effect size for confounding variables or differences in length of follow-up. For example, in a cohort study of the predictors of hip fractures, you can determine the effect of family history of fracture after adjusting for age, sex, and history of falls.

Logistic regression models are used when the time to the outcome is not known or does not matter. In a study of the predictors of in-hospital survival after a sudden cardiac arrest, you would use logistic regression models because the research question implies that a death on day 2 of the hospitalization is the same as a death on Day 5. Hazard models are used when the time to the event matters and is known. Proportional hazards models are also useful when the amount of follow-up varies among the subjects. This can happen, for example, if subjects were enrolled at different times or if many subjects dropped out or died of unrelated causes during follow-up. Logistic regression models yield odds ratios; proportional hazards models yield rate (hazard) ratios.

If you have used one of these more complex models, ask your biostatistician to tell you the odds ratio (or rate ratio) for each variable that interests you. Make sure that you understand the definition of the predictor and the outcome variables, the units being compared, the direction of the effect, and how to express the regression coefficient as a clinically meaningful effect. For example, it is useless to be told that "the logistic regression coefficient for glucose was 0.0034." You need to know that the predictor variable was baseline glucose level measured in mg per dL, that the outcome variable was defined as having pneumonia during 2 years of follow-up, and that the regression coefficient was defined per mg per dL increase in glucose level. All this corresponds to an odds ratio of developing pneumonia of 1.4 per 100 mg/dL increase.

Another common type of analysis is called *survival analysis,* which often has nothing to do with living or dying. The word survival, often referred to as disease-free survival, refers to the concept of remaining free of the outcome of interest, and it is used irrespective of whether the outcome is fatal or not. In a study of gout, for example, a disease-free survival of 2 years means that the subject did not develop gout during 2 years of follow-up.

Usually, survival curves show the proportions of subjects free of the event (on the *y*-axis), by time (on the *x*-axis), in different groups. Survival curves might compare event-free survival in the intervention group and the control group in a clinical trial, or by different stages of disease. Survival curves usually include the denominators of subjects without the outcome remaining in the study at each important time point (e.g., at baseline and every 6 months in a 2-year study).

Survival analysis is especially useful when everyone, or nearly everyone in the study, either gets better or gets worse. Then, what matters is how quickly that happens. For example, when evaluating a new treatment for common cold, comparing the time to recovery in the treatment and control groups makes much more sense than comparing the proportion who were better at 1 month. After all, no matter how good the treatment was, just about everyone in the control group would have recovered by then. In a study of a new treatment for pancreatic cancer, comparing the survival curves in the treatment and control groups would be more useful than comparing the proportion who were alive at 5 years. In these situations, the effect size is usually the difference in median time to recovery for conditions that usually resolve or to death for conditions that are usually fatal.

Effect Sizes for Dichotomous Predictors and Continuous Outcome Variables

Usually, this sort of effect size comes from a study that compares two groups, say, the treatment group and the control group in a clinical trial. What should be compared? The means in the two groups? The medians? The distributions in the two groups? In part, this depends on the shape of the distribution of the outcome variable. So long as the shape is close to "normal" or at least is reasonably symmetric, the means can be compared, and the effect size is the difference in the means. If the shape is not normal, then the usual choice is to compare the entire distributions in the two groups using nonparametric statistics, explained in the section "Where Do *P* Values Come From?" in this chapter. As there is no convenient effect size for comparing distributions, you usually also provide the median values in the two groups, perhaps along with the 25th and 75th (or 10th and 90th) percentiles.

When comparing means, should you use the absolute difference (e.g., 8 mm Hg of systolic blood pressure [SBP]) or the percentage difference (e.g., a 5% difference)? This is a situation in which putting one of the comparisons in a table (or figure) and the other in the text may be the best solution. Certainly, if the measurement and its units are not familiar to readers, then the percentage difference will be friendlier.

For studies that involve making multiple measurements of the same variable in each subject, the big decision involves choosing the outcome variable. Should it be the final value of the outcome variable (e.g., urate level at 1 year) or the change in that variable during the study (change in urate level from baseline to the final value)? If you choose to compare the change in a variable during a study, remember that the primary comparison should be between groups rather than within groups.

Effect Sizes for Continuous Predictor Variables and Continuous Outcome Variables

On occasion, an effect size may involve the association between two continuous variables. In this sort of situation, the linear regression slope—the change in the outcome per unit change in the predictor—is the simplest effect size to understand. For example, in a study of the effect of age on cognitive function in the elderly, the effect size might be that each 1-year increase in age is associated with a 0.6-point decline in cognitive function. (*Note*: This is the same as saying that each 5-year increase in age is associated with a 3-point decline, or each 10 years with a 6-point decline. The choice as to whether to use 1 year, 5 years, or 10 years is somewhat arbitrary; my preference is to use a value that spans roughly one-quarter of the range in the sample. So if your sample ranged in age from 65 to 90 years, then 5 years would be a good choice.)

The commonest type of regression involves assuming that two variables are related in a linear fashion:

$$\text{Continuous outcome} = \text{slope} \times (\text{continuous predictor}) + \text{intercept}$$

For example,

$$\text{Cognitive function} = -0.6 \times \text{age} + 50$$

The minus sign indicates that as age increases, cognitive function decreases. There are other types of regression that involve, for example, determining the relation between the outcome and the square of the predictor variable or the log of the predictor.

An alternative is to use the correlation between the predictor and outcome variables, which is easy to estimate. Correlations vary from −1 to +1. A correlation of 0 indicates that there is no association between the variables; correlations close to 1 (or −1) indicate that the two variables are closely related in a linear fashion; therefore knowing the value of one of the variables provides a lot of information about the other variable.

There is a simple (albeit obscure if you have never taken statistics) relation between the correlation coefficient (r), the linear regression slope, the standard deviation of the predictor variable (SD_p), and the outcome variable (SD_o):

$$r = \frac{\text{Slope} \times SD_p}{SD_o}$$

The square of a correlation coefficient (r^2) yields the proportion of the variance (spread) in one variable that is explained by the other variable. For example, if level of education is correlated with family income at $r = 0.9$, then 81% of the spread in income levels is explained by differences in education. However, you cannot assume that one of the variables causes the other; it is just as correct to say that much of the spread in educational level is explained by differences in income.

A correlation of 0.3, which corresponds to only 9% of the variance explained, does not sound very impressive: 91% of the variance is unexplained. But for many variables, there is a lot of "random noise" in the measurement, or a lot of other factors that also matter, so explaining 9% of the variance may be all that you can expect.

STATISTICS

"Real" statistics—the stuff that yields confidence intervals and P values—constitute the fourth step in presenting results, in that they demonstrate the precision of your effect sizes.

Indicating the Precision of an Estimate with a Confidence Interval

The *confidence interval* for a point estimate is the range of values that are consistent with that estimate. Confidence intervals can be used to indicate the precision of descriptive results such as proportions or means or of analytic results such as risk ratios and risk differences. Confidence intervals are enormously important. A risk ratio of 10 for the association between gum chewing and tongue cancer sounds pretty impressive, but if it is based on only a few outcomes, and therefore has a confidence interval from 0.5 to 200, the point estimate of 10 has very little meaning. That estimate is consistent with the possibility that chewing gum is associated with a 50% lower, or 200 times greater, risk of tongue cancer. Conversely, a risk ratio of 10 with a confidence interval from 8 to 13 has a great deal of meaning. In that situation, gum chewing is definitely associated with a substantial increase in risk. Whether it is an 8-fold increase, a 10-fold increase, or a 13-fold increase is not likely to matter very much.

To this point, the discussion of confidence intervals has been oversimplified because a phrase has been left out. There is no such thing as a "confidence interval" per se. You must always refer to an $X\%$ confidence interval, usually the 95% confidence interval. The "95%" has a misleadingly simple explanation: It implies that if you repeat a bias-free study many times, 95% of all the confidence intervals for the point estimate will contain the true value in the population. (Unfortunately, that does not mean that any particular 95% confidence interval has a 95% chance of containing the true value. For example, if you have a strange finding, such as a 95% confidence interval of 0.3 to 0.7 for the relative risk of lung cancer in smokers, that does not mean that you would be 95% sure that smoking actually protects against lung cancer.)

The wider a confidence interval, the less precise is the point estimate. A mean creatinine clearance of 70 mL/minute, with a 95% confidence interval from 65 to 75 mL/minute, is a more precise estimate than if the 95% confidence intervals reached from 50 to 90 mL/minute. Usually, a narrower interval indicates a larger sample size, but it may also indicate a better measurement method. Sloppy measurements lead to wide confidence intervals.

Most commonly, you will use 95% confidence intervals. But you can use others, such as a 90% confidence interval, which will make the confidence interval much narrower, or a 99% confidence interval, which will make it much wider.

Confidence intervals are bell shaped, not bar shaped. That is, values at the ends of a confidence interval, near the upper and lower bounds, are less likely than values near the middle.

Confidence intervals are symmetric about the point estimate. The 95% confidence interval extends approximately from two standard errors below to two standard errors above the point estimate.

Lower bound of 95% confidence interval ≈ point estimate − 2 × standard error of point estimate

Upper bound of 95% confidence interval ≈ point estimate + 2 × standard error of point estimate

However, for point estimates that involve division (such as odds ratios and rate ratios), the confidence interval is estimated on a different scale, so that the confidence interval is symmetric about the log of the point estimate. This makes determining the 95% confidence interval for these types of point estimates trickier; the method is discussed in the Appendix.

So far, the process of determining a 95% confidence interval simply involves determining the standard error of your point estimate. Fortunately, most statistical programs, if they have not provided the 95% confidence interval, do provide the standard error. And as was mentioned earlier in the chapter, for a continuous measurement, the standard error of the mean is simply $SD \div \sqrt{N}$, where N equals the number of measurements.

Actually, the process of determining a confidence interval also involves knowing whether 2 is the right number to use. In most circumstances, 1.96 is the actual value for 95% confidence intervals, and, given the lack of precision in your estimate of the standard error, using 2 will work just fine. All standard statistical books provide enough information to figure out the real values to use. This matters more when the sample size is small, for example, <30. These books also provide the values to use to determine the 90% or 99% confidence interval, or any other value you choose.

Although confidence intervals are usually used with analytic results, on occasion a descriptive result is important enough to warrant having a confidence interval.

In a survey of 1,283 randomly selected Americans, 31% (95% confidence interval: 26% to 36%) reported that they believed in evolution, whereas only 29% (95% confidence interval: 24% to 34%) believed in the tooth fairy.

P Values and Confidence Intervals

With analytic results, many investigators are accustomed to determining the *P* value to see whether the result is statistically significant. Setting aside the meaning of statistical significance and *P* values discussed below, there is a straightforward relation between *P* values and confidence intervals. Understanding that relation requires the concept of *no effect,* an analytic result that indicates no difference between the groups being compared. For effect sizes that involve subtraction (e.g., mean difference) and for slopes and correlations, *no effect* is an effect size of 0. For effect sizes that involve division (e.g., risk ratios), *no effect* is an effect size of 1. Examples of *no effect* are provided in Table 5.3.

A 95% confidence interval that excludes *no effect* implies that the *P* value will be <0.05. For example, suppose the mean difference in serum bicarbonate levels between two groups is 5 mEq/L with a 95% confidence interval from 2 to 8 mEq/L. That confidence interval excludes *no effect* (zero difference, or 0 mEg/L). Therefore, the two groups are significantly different at $P < 0.05$. If either the upper or lower bound for a 95% confidence interval exactly equals *no effect,* then the *P* value is exactly 0.05. For example, if the relative risk of osteosarcoma in smokers is 2.0, with a 95% confidence interval from 1.0 to 4.0, it means that the *P* value is 0.05. Finally, if a 95% confidence interval includes *no effect,* then the *P* value must be >0.05. If *no effect* lies close to the middle of a 95% confidence interval, then the *P* value will be much >0.05. For example, if an odds ratio is 1.4, with a 95% confidence interval from 0.5 to 4, then the *P* value is substantially >0.05.

TABLE 5.3	Examples of No Effect
Effect Size Measured	**No Effect**
Difference in prevalence	0
Risk difference	0
Rate difference	0
Number needed to treat	∞
Mean difference	0
Mean percentage difference	0
Mean change	0
Mean percentage change	0
Slope	0
Correlation	0
Prevalence ratio	1
Risk ratio	1
Odds ratio	1
Rate ratio (or hazard ratio)	1

More generally, an X% confidence interval is the range of results that would not differ statistically from the point estimate at $P = (100 - X)/100$.

What Do Statistical Significance and Differ Statistically Actually Mean?

Statistical significance is somewhat counterintuitive. Rather than trying to show that something is probably happening, you try to show that it is improbable that something is not happening. You assume that there is nothing going on, then look for evidence to the contrary. How do you do this? The basic idea is that if there were really no effect, then certain results—for example, those that show a big effect—should not happen. So, if you find a big effect, then it is unlikely that nothing was going on.

The problem is that big effects can sometimes happen by chance. Suppose, for example, that you have been asked to determine whether a coin has been altered to come up heads more often than tails. In this situation, *no effect* implies that the proportions of heads and tails should be equal. You flip the coin twice, and it comes up heads both times. Would you conclude that this was an unfair coin? Probably not, because even a fair coin will sometimes (25% of the time, of course) come up two heads in a row. What if four consecutive tosses come up heads? Once again, that hardly constitutes very strong evidence against the coin being fair. Although 100% of the tosses were heads, four heads in a row happens 6.3% of the time. But if the coin were tossed 1,000 times and came up heads on 550 of them, that would be strong evidence against the coin being fair because with a fair coin, getting 550 or more heads would happen <0.2% of the time.

In statistical terminology, *no effect* is called the *null hypothesis*. The process of deciding that it is unlikely that there is no effect is known as *rejecting the null hypothesis*. The ability to reject a null hypothesis has been made possible by generations of statisticians, who have figured out what might happen for all sorts of null hypotheses and have then determined the likelihood of various results.

The process yields what is called a P value, which is the chance that a result as extreme as the one that was observed (or even more extreme) would have been observed under the null hypothesis. If that chance is <5%, you say that the result was statistically significant at $P < 0.05$. If that chance is <0.1%, you say that the result was statistically significant at $P < 0.001$. But, if the result was close to *no effect* (e.g., 498 of 1,000 tosses being heads), or if the sample was small (4 coin tosses), then the P value will be >0.05.

A big study with a relatively small effect size can still have a significant P value. For example, if a coin is tossed 10,000 times and 51% of the tosses are heads, then it is unlikely that the coin is fair. But it is not unfair by very much. In fact, a P value of 0.05 in a small study implies a larger effect size than the same P value in a bigger study.

Freedom from the Tyranny of 0.05

There is, however, nothing magical about the value 0.05, despite its illustrious history and omnipresence in statistics. Why should a result that has a P value of 0.049 be important, whereas one with a P value of 0.051, or even 0.07, is meaningless? A

P value of 0.001 is much less likely under the null hypothesis than a *P* value of 0.04. Those are two reasons why actual *P* values, rather than just <0.05 or nonsignificant (NS) should be provided.

It is simply silly to regard as "nonsignificant" results that have *P* values that are barely >0.05 or 95% confidence intervals that barely overlap *no effect*. Many also realize that it is just as silly to accept as gospel those results that have *P* values that are just barely <0.05, or 95% confidence intervals that barely miss *no effect*. Alas, the same cannot be said for all-too-many reviewers and even some journal editors.

The best course of action depends on whether results with a *P* value that is "right around 0.05" make sense. If the results seem odd, or inconsistent with previous work, then chance is a likely explanation, and you should say so. If the results are consistent with other studies, or make good sense, then results with *P* values close to 0.05 are more likely to reflect a real difference between the groups that were compared.

Most investigators are concerned about reporting a study that does not have any *P* values <0.05, a so-called negative study. They succumb to the temptation to dredge through their data until they can find some combination of predictors and outcomes, or some subgroup of the sample, that will yield a result with a significant *P* value. Please do not do this.

Why not? Because if you have designed and executed your study carefully, then the absence of any statistically significant results should not hurt its publication prospects. What you must do in that situation, however, is explain carefully why your "negative" results matter. That argument hinges on using confidence intervals to turn a liability—no significant *P* values—into a strength. You do this by ruling out important effects. Because the 95% confidence intervals for your key results overlap *no effect* if the *P* values are >0.05, then the sole remaining question is, how far do they extend in either direction around *no effect*? Is the confidence interval sufficiently narrow, as it should be in a well-designed study, to exclude the possibility that you missed a clinically important effect?

For example, suppose you compare the risk of peptic ulcer disease in people with high-stress jobs to the risk in people in low-stress occupations and find that the risk ratio is 0.9 with a 95% confidence interval from 0.7 to 1.2. This is good evidence that job stress is not an important cause of peptic ulcer disease. You would have a more difficult time convincing reviewers that your results were meaningful, however, if the point estimate was 0.9, with a 95% confidence interval from 0.2 to 4.0. The upper limit of your confidence interval includes the possibility of a substantial effect of job stress on the risk of ulcers.

Even with a narrow confidence interval, convincing manuscript reviewers and journal editors can sometimes be difficult with a negative study. Even the most statistically literate reviewers may not be willing to get beyond an innate tendency to reject a manuscript if the *P* value for the main result is >0.05. If this happens—and if you are a clinical investigator for long enough, it will—perhaps it will be of some comfort to realize that you are joining a club with many other, equally frustrated, members.

That said, results with confidence intervals that overlap *no effect* or nonsignificant *P* values are not always meaningful. A poorly designed and poorly executed study is likely to be negative. Noisy measurements, dropouts, or poorly defined predictor or outcome variables make it harder to find effects, even if they are real.

Precision of Effect Sizes, Confidence Intervals, and *P* Values

Just as with descriptive results, the precision of an effect size should be consistent with the number of subjects and events. With 20 events, a risk ratio (RR) is 2.0, not 2.023, and the *P* value will be 0.4, not 0.365. Similarly, it is absurd to report, "The RR was 2.023 with a 95% confidence interval from 1.031 to 3.969." Just say, "The RR was 2.0 with a 95% confidence interval from 1.0 to 4.0." If you are concerned that a reviewer will think that the results are NS because the confidence interval touches 1.0, then include the *P* value:

> The RR of lymphoma was 2.0 with a 95% confidence interval from 1.0 to 4.0 (*P* = 0.04).

This sort of attention to numerical detail will help you recognize the limitations of your data and thereby avoid the mistake of emphasizing the difference between 36.4% and 42.9% when you were actually comparing 4 of 11 with 3 of 7.

P values rarely need to be more precise than the nearest 0.01 (e.g., 0.43, not 0.4273, or 0.04, not 0.0395), unless they are <0.01, in which case using <0.001 or <0.0001 is adequate. A *P* value of 0.0000001 (or $P < 10^{-7}$) is overkill. When *P* values get very small, the issue is rarely whether the results are very, very, very statistically significant or unbelievably statistically significant. The usual issue is whether the results are real or result from bias or some other design or analysis flaw. The exception, of course, involves some genetic studies (like genome-wide association studies), in which statistical significance is set at very low levels because so many (literally tens of thousands or more) different effect sizes are being tested.

Comparing *P* Values

One of the great temptations of clinical research is to compare two *P* values—one for a statistically significant result and the other for a result that was not statistically significant—and state that this pair of *P* values implies that the two groups are different. *Do not do this.* For example, suppose a study finds that men lost weight on a high-fiber diet (*P* < 0.03), whereas women did not (*P* = 0.45). The temptation is to conclude that the diet works in men, but not in women. That would be wrong. The way to test whether such a conclusion is statistically meaningful would be to determine the mean difference between the changes in weight in men and in women and ascertain whether that difference was statistically different from zero.

Where Do *P* Values Come from?

Calculating *P* values is not difficult. Most of the time, you simply divide the effect size by its standard error and look up the result (the "standardized" effect size) in a table. The type of table to be used depends on the type of statistical test, which in turn depends on the type of predictor and outcome variables. The table tells you how likely it is that such a standardized effect, or one even larger, would happen by chance under the null hypothesis. For example, if you are comparing the mean value in two groups using Student's *t* test, then:

$$t = \frac{\text{Difference in means}}{\text{Standard error of the difference}}$$

Other, roughly equivalent, formulas exist. There are a few important exceptions to this general formula. One involves the comparison of dichotomous predictors and dichotomous outcomes. Determining the P value for these comparisons involves using the χ^2 test or Fisher's exact test. (Although the χ^2- test is easier to understand and certainly easier to calculate, Fisher's exact test should be used whenever the sample size is small, for example, if any of the numbers are less than about five.)

Another exception is *analysis of variance,* or ANOVA, which is a statistical technique to determine whether several means are different from one another. The technique is called ANOVA because the methodology involves looking at the spread (variance) of the values in a continuous variable and determining how much of that spread results from a categorical variable. For example, you could perform an ANOVA of the effects of blood type on hemoglobin concentration. If the mean hemoglobin values are very different by blood type, then much of the spread of hemoglobin values in the sample will be because of blood type. ANOVA should be used to show that differences among mean values in several groups are greater than what would be expected by chance. However, ANOVA would not tell you which of the blood types were mainly responsible for the different hemoglobin values; that would require comparing the mean values between individual blood types using t tests. It would be a mistake to start with t tests, however, because you can easily pick out the two groups that have the biggest difference to compare. Only if there are significant differences among all the groups should you look for differences between any of the pairs of groups.

More sophisticated ANOVA techniques allow you to look at repeated measurements in the same individual, to see if there are differences in those values at different times. For example, investigators conducting a 3-year study of the effect of two diets on cognitive function could use ANOVA to determine whether the diets had any effect, whether time had any effect (did subjects get worse?), and even whether the effects of the diets varied at different times.

Another important exception involves what are called *nonparametric distributions*. They are called *nonparametric* because they cannot be described by specific parameters, such as a mean and a SD—the way a t distribution, an F distribution, or a χ^2 distribution can. If you find that distinction unhelpful, then all you really need to know about the most commonly used nonparametric statistics is that the exact values being compared do not matter, only their rank. For example, in comparing the value of an outcome variable (say, IQ score) in two groups using a nonparametric test, you simply record the group with the highest value, one with the next highest value, and so on. Under the null hypothesis, those ranks should be distributed by chance in the two groups. If it turns out, however, that one group has many more of the high-ranking values than the other, it is unlikely to have occurred by chance under the null hypothesis, and you would say that the two distributions are different.

Nonparametric distributions are particularly useful for skewed data (those whose distribution does not look even vaguely bell shaped), such as length of stay. They are also useful if you want to avoid placing undue emphasis on a single value or two. For example, in a study of income in two groups, one subject with a celebrity entertainer type of income will make the mean income in his group unusually high. A nonparametric comparison would minimize the impact of that income.

Multivariable Techniques

Up to this point in the chapter, the effect size has meant the effect of variable A on variable B. Multivariable techniques allow the determination of the effect of A on B after adjusting for C (D, E, etc.). There are scores of different multivariable techniques available, including linear regression, analysis of covariance, logistic regression, and proportional hazards models. The trade-off is that the effect size, instead of being something simple to understand, such as a mean difference or a risk ratio, tends to be more complicated, such as a regression coefficient. These models assess the statistical significance of their results by comparing the regression coefficient with its standard error. Fortunately, you can usually convert the regression coefficient to a more familiar estimate, such as an odds ratio, hazard ratio, or slope.

Because the models tend to have a bit of black-box quality to them—you select a few tests on the computer and out pops the regression coefficient and a P value—try not to present just the "modeled" results. If possible, provide the actual data. For example, if one of your key findings is the correlation between two variables (body mass index and serum high-density lipoprotein cholesterol levels), do not just present the correlation or the regression equation. Include the scatter plot, along with the regression line.

If you used a sophisticated analytic technique, such as logistic regression or proportional hazards models, your statistical analyst (or your computer program) may have handed you a list of "significant" (and NS) results. How can these be interpreted? (The same general ideas that are discussed here can also be applied to models for continuous outcome variables.)

In a study of the risk factors for oral cancer, for example, you may have found that age, alcohol use, cigarette smoking, and number of sexual partners were statistically significant predictors. How was this determination made? If you did not do this analysis yourself, you need to understand that these techniques are not automatic. Many decisions were made before the computer disgorged the answer. Be sure that you agree with these decisions. It is important to understand that this is not a passive process. An analyst must specify a single dichotomous outcome variable (e.g., developed oral cancer during the study), develop a list of potential predictor variables to be examined (e.g., age in years, sex, race, body weight, cigarette smoking in pack-years, number of sexual partners, history of alcohol abuse, history of dental caries, etc.), determine the statistical criterion for including a variable in the model, and choose the order in which variables are considered. Some analysts also verify that the assumptions in the model, which determine the validity of the algorithm that the computer uses, are reasonable. With all those options, giving the same data set to two analysts with instructions to "analyze the data" may lead to two different sets of results.

One assumption in most models is that the relation between a continuous predictor variable and the outcome variable is the same for all values of the predictor. For example, a logistic regression model with age as a continuous variable assumes that the effects of a 1-year increase in age are the same when comparing 1-year-old with 2-year-old children as when comparing 69-year-old with 70-year-old adults. When this assumption is not valid, such as if there is a U-shaped or threshold relation between the predictor and the outcome, the model will also not be valid.

If you did not do the analysis yourself, ask your analyst which predictor variables were tested in the models. What criteria were used to determine whether a potential risk factor was included in, or excluded from, the final model? Get a list of the variables that were checked and find out how the analyst decided which ones would be in the final model. Were models built by adding variables one at a time to identify those that mattered? Or did the analyst start with a lot of variables and subtract those that did not matter? What statistical criteria were used to determine whether to include a variable in the model (say, $P < 0.05$ or <0.10) or exclude a variable? Were some variables forced into the models? How were the predictor variables analyzed? Was age treated as a continuous variable (age in years), as a categorical variable (by 10-year age groups), or as a dichotomous variable (<50 years of age, ≥50 years)?

How should continuous variables be categorized or dichotomized? If there is a logical way to split a variable, then do it that way. Measurements of thyroid-stimulating hormone might be classified as low, normal, or high based on the normal range in the laboratory. SBP might be categorized as ≤119 mm Hg, 120 to 139 mm Hg, 140 to 159 mm Hg, and ≥160 mm Hg.

Another categorization option is to divide a variable by percentiles—for example, by quartiles or quintiles. One advantage of doing this is that the sample size is equal in each category. Another benefit is that you can divide several measurements, such as blood pressure, serum cholesterol, and vitamin B_{12} levels, the same way. The chief disadvantage is that the values in the percentiles are likely to vary from one study to another, which makes it difficult to compare the results in different studies. In addition, the differences in the spread of values of the predictor variable from one percentile to the next may vary considerably.

How many data were missing? In a multivariable model, a subject who is missing data on any of the variables is eliminated from the model, unless special techniques of estimating or imputing the missing data are used.

Special Issues: Model Fit and Interactions

In the end, the analysis will select a single "best-fitting" model given the variables that were examined and the chosen modeling technique. But that model may not fit much better than other models, some of which may make more clinical or biologic sense. Were models that used a different set of variables also tried? How much difference did changing the variables make? Try to avoid hanging your hat on a single, final model that explains everything. An alternative model, or perhaps several, probably works almost as well.

How closely did the model fit the actual data? One simple test involves comparing what the model predicts should happen with what actually happened. For a dichotomous outcome, was the actual risk the lowest among subjects whom the model had predicted to be at the lowest risk? Did the model perform well across all risk groups, such as those predicted to be at high, moderate, or low risk?

Another vexing issue is whether to look for interactions in your analysis. An interaction means that the effects of a predictor variable on the outcome depend on another variable. For example, the effects of serum cholesterol on mortality appear to depend on age. In young people, the higher the cholesterol level, the higher the mortality rate, whereas in older persons, the association between cholesterol and mortality flattens out. However, interactions are rare biologically, usually hard to detect, and almost always difficult to understand, although it does not prevent many investigators from trying.

There are two main ways to deal with interactions. First, you can present the different associations between the primary predictor variable and the outcome separately in different categories of the other variable. Thus, the association between cholesterol and mortality could be presented for subjects stratified by age into groups of younger than 40 years old, 40 to 59 years old, 60 to 79 years old, and 80 years and older. The chief advantage of this method is ease of explanation; the main problem is that the sample size may get small in each of the strata. Second, you can introduce what is called an *interaction term* into the model, to measure the effect of the interaction and to determine whether it is statistically significant (most are not and represent noise or overanalysis of the data). In the example, the interaction term might be a new variable that equaled age in years multiplied by cholesterol level. For reasons that are not worth going into here, including this term along with age and cholesterol in the analyses often works. Although this strategy preserves the size of the sample, it is always difficult to explain the meaning of a statistically significant interaction term to readers.

WHAT READERS WILL EXPECT TO FIND

Now that you know the way to present your point estimates and their precision, what actually belongs in a Results section, and in what order? There are certain basic categories that nearly every manuscript should include.

Descriptive Results

Start by describing who was in your study, including demographic characteristics such as sex, age, and race; clinical characteristics such as medical history, habits, and current medications; and key predictor variables, whatever these are in your study. This allows readers to determine to whom your results apply. Often, these results are presented in a table, commonly separated by the groups that are being compared (e.g., treatment vs. placebo group; cases vs. controls). See Chapter 6 for specific instructions on how to format tables describing study participants.

You should also tell readers about your outcome variable, so they know what happened in your study. If your outcome variable was dichotomous, such as *developed cervical cancer or not,* then you should tell how many subjects had the outcome. If your outcome variable was continuous, such as *change in insulin levels,* or *24-hour urinary protein excretion at 6 weeks,* then you should describe it. If you followed subjects for a specific period, that should also be mentioned:

> We enrolled 234 subjects who were followed for 90 days following initial hospital discharge.
>
> During that time, 67 (29%) were readmitted. Most of the patients were elderly women with chronic medical problems (Table 1).
>
> Data were available for 67 patients with myasthenia gravis who had been treated with immunosuppressive therapy, of whom 52 (78%) had anticholinesterase antibody titers of 1:64 or greater.

During an average of 4 years of follow-up, mean fasting glucose levels had increased by 35 mg per dL. Of the 260 subjects who were alive at the end of follow-up, 36 (14%) developed evidence of nephropathy.

The characteristics you present should correspond to the analytic results that you will soon mention. If, for example, you are going to present analytic data on the association between current use of hormone replacement therapy and pulmonary embolism in women, then be sure you also provide the proportion of women currently using hormone replacement. Do not just provide the proportion of women who have ever used hormone replacement, the mean number of years of use, or the average dose among users.

In general, the characteristics of the subjects are descriptive of those who were enrolled in the study, even if not all of them remained in the study. However, if there were many subjects who had dropped out, or for whom there were missing data, you should also indicate how the final sample differed from the original sample. In a randomized trial, the fundamental rule is *once randomized, always analyzed.* That is, the main description should be of the original groups, including their baseline characteristics and what happened to them in the study. In a cohort or cross-sectional study, describe the entire sample; if there are important subsamples, such as men and women, describe them. In a case–control study, describe the cases and the controls. In a study of a diagnostic or prognostic test, describe those with the outcome (disease) and the controls.

Main Finding

Next, present your basic analytic findings, with few details. Make sure the effect size is crystal clear:

During an average of 6 years of follow-up, survival was 9% (95% confidence interval: 4% to 14%; $P < 0.001$) greater among subjects treated with novastatin than in the control group (Figure 1). Approximately four of five novastatin patients, compared with 70% of control patients, survived for 5 or more years.

Subjects with anticholinesterase antibodies were twice as likely (95% confidence interval, 1.2 to 3.3) to respond to immunosuppressive therapy.

Remember these three basic tenets: (1) do not bury the main findings at the middle or end of a paragraph where no one will notice them; (2) do not obscure them by using fancy statistical terms; and (3) do not forget the effect size.

Buried Findings:

We followed the subjects for an average of 2 months (range 1 to 6 months); follow-up was 98% complete. Using an intention-to-treat analysis, adjusting for baseline differences in the groups in age, serum LDH level, and history of alcohol use, we found ....

Obscured Findings:

Factor analysis disclosed that eigenvalues were significant for the cognitive and social domains.

Forgotten Effect Size:

There were statistically significant differences between the two groups.

Not all key findings must be positive results, in the sense of having a statistically significant association. Important negative results, along with their confidence intervals, should be included in the manuscript.

Other Important Findings

After presenting the main results, mention the consistency of results within the study, using alternate definitions of variables or in important subgroups:

Whether we defined hypertension using diastolic, systolic, or mean blood pressures, the results were similar.

Looking at arrhythmias that occurred in the first 24 hours, we found that the use of digoxin was associated with a reduced risk of atrial fibrillation. Similar results were seen during the first 72 hours.

The effects were similar in men and in women, and by major age categories (<45, 46 to 55, and >55 years).

If more elaborate statistical models were used, then discuss them:

Adjusting for age, race, sex, and family income in multivariable logistic regression models did not affect these results.

This segment of the Results section can also include additional supporting evidence, including alternative measurement methods, different analytic techniques, and analyses in various subgroups. These can sometimes be included in the same paragraph as the main finding, particularly, if they pertain to a variant of the key predictor or outcome variable:

Rates of myocardial infarction were about two fold greater in the control group. This was also true for stroke and heart failure.

Whether we used the standard method of measuring antibody titers, or the new technique developed in our laboratory, the results were the same.

Additional Results

Additional results include material that may not be part of the main story. This might include more elaborate questions, such as estimated cost-effectiveness of an intervention, or experimental or pilot results in a few subjects. End the Results section with any surprising findings that seem important to mention. If these results do not have enough bulk to warrant a separate publication (perhaps a letter to the editor), it may be worthwhile to include them in the main manuscript. But be prepared to eliminate them if requested to do so by an editor trying to save space.

GETTING STARTED

If you are having a hard time with the Results section of your manuscript, go back to your list of key results. Write about them as if your target audience consisted of 10-year-old children:

> Most of the people ($n = 87$) in our study were young men and women who came to the emergency room with broken ankles; a few were referred directly from the office of an orthopedic surgeon ($n = 6$) or podiatrist ($n = 3$). Usually, the fractures were the result of a fall.

Ultimately, settle on language that an educated person with an interest in science can understand. You will be pleasantly surprised how closely that resembles your first draft for children.

Important: Read This Section

Many beginning investigators make the mistake of writing their Results section around their tables and figures. The resulting manuscript reads like a boring tour of an art museum.

> Picture 1 is by van Gogh. That sculpture is by Matisse. The next painting was painted in 1904.

> Table 1 shows … . Figure 1 demonstrates … . The multivariate results can be seen in Table 2. … Figure 2 is the survival curve.

Although there is nothing intrinsically awful about this type of writing, it violates a key rule, that the text, tables, and figures should complement one another. What does *complement* mean? If the table provides the participants' mean weights and cholesterol levels and the proportions of who had diabetes and hypertension, then you might say this in the text:

> Participants were generally obese with a high prevalence of cardiovascular risk factors (Table 2).

If the table includes the mean age of the participants, you might mention in the text that 30% of the subjects were older than 65 years of age. If the results in the table were presented separately for men and women, then present some of the overall results in the text.

Ideally, the text highlights the tables and figures by suggesting that the reader look for a particular finding or compare the results in different figures. Try to imitate a knowledgeable docent in an art museum:

> On the far wall, van Gogh uses brush strokes to convey the emotional content of a landscape. By contrast, the neighboring canvas by Matisse relies on color alone to convey mood. Notice how weightless Degas makes the ballet dancer appear.

> By contrast with the clear association between greater cholesterol level and mortality in persons younger than 55 years of age (Figure 1), there was little association in older persons (Figure 2).

When you provide this sort of docent-like guidance, the reader knows what to expect and can interpret your table (or figure) more easily.

If there are lots of numbers in your text, and the exact values matter, then a table will be appropriate. If the exact values are less important than the pattern or trends in the data, then a figure will be a better choice. As the Results section takes shape, the need for additional tables or figures, or the possibility of eliminating a few, may become evident. See Chapters 6 and 7 on tables and figures for additional guidance.

If you still cannot organize the results clearly, use subheads. These may not be a permanent part of the manuscript, but they may help you as you write a draft. Here are some examples:

What Happened to Subjects

Results in Men Compared with Women

Multivariable Models

Long-Term Follow-Up

Quality-of-Life Measurements

Effects of O_2 Supplementation

Comparison of Responders and Nonresponders

✓ CHECKLIST FOR

THE RESULTS SECTION

1. Did you provide the basic results of the study (e.g., how many lived, how many died, and the key descriptive characteristics)?

2. Are the effect sizes for the main outcomes of the study easy to find?

3. Does the text complement the tables and figures?

4. Is the level of precision for descriptive and analytic results appropriate to the sample size?

5. Are unusual or surprising results in their proper place?

Reference

1. Newman TB, Browner WS, Cummings SR. Designing studies of medical tests. In: Hulley SB, Cummings SR, Browner WS, et al., eds. *Designing Clinical Research: An Epidemiologic Approach*. 3rd ed. Philadelphia, PA: Lippincott Williams & Wilkins; 2007.

A

Appendix: Converting Regression Coefficients into Clinically Meaningful Terms

Throughout this appendix, the example refers to the logistic regression model, which is based on the odds of an event and the odds ratio associated with a predictor variable. The same principles hold for the Cox proportional hazards model, except that the model looks at the rate of an event and the rate ratio.

Along with understanding how to convert a regression coefficient from a logistic model into an odds ratio, it is also worthwhile knowing where those coefficients came from. That, however, is beyond the scope of this book. For our purposes, it is enough to say that a computer algorithm selects the values. For each predictor variable in the model, the "computer" generates a regression coefficient per unit increase of that variable, along with a standard error for that coefficient. The regression coefficient is called b, or sometimes β. It needs to be exponentiated (raised to the power of e) to yield an odds ratio:

$$\text{Odds ratio} = e^b$$

Before this is done, however, you need to know the unit and direction of change that the coefficient refers to. For example, suppose the regression coefficient is 0.4 for the risk of stroke from smoking. Does that mean current smokers were compared with nonsmokers? Or that ex-smokers were compared with people who had never smoked? Or does the coefficient of 0.4 refer to, say, each 10-pack-year increase in smoking history?

Assume that the comparison is between current smokers and nonsmokers. Then, a regression coefficient of 0.4 for stroke means:

$$\text{OR (current smokers vs. nonsmokers)} = e^{0.4} = 1.5$$

In other words, the odds of stroke are 1.5-fold higher in current smokers than in nonsmokers.

What about a categorical predictor variable, such as activity on a 1 (very sedentary) to 5 (very active) scale? In that case, the regression coefficient represents the effect of a one-unit increase in activity. Therefore, a regression coefficient of 0.2 for activity and stroke implies:

$$\text{OR per one-unit increase in activity} = e^{0.2} = 1.25$$

Therefore, each one-unit change in activity is associated with 25% greater odds of stroke. This assumes that the odds of having a stroke increase in a "log-linear" fashion (each change, such as from category 1 [very sedentary] to category 2 [sedentary], or from category 3 [average] to category 4 [active], has the same effect). If this assumption is not true, then you need to treat each of the different activity categories as separate variables (and use something called "dummy" variables in your analyses: Ask your statistician for help on this).

What about a continuous predictor variable, such as diastolic blood pressure (DBP)? A regression coefficient of 0.01 for the association between DBP in mm Hg and stroke implies:

$$\text{OR per 1 mm Hg increase in DBP} = e^{0.01} = 1.01$$

Therefore, a 1 mm Hg increase in blood pressure is associated with 1% greater odds of stroke. For a continuous variable, this is not particularly useful because we are rarely interested in a one-unit change. Fortunately, there is a simple way to determine the odds ratio for stroke associated with, say, a 20 mm Hg increase in DBP. You simply multiply the regression coefficient by the amount of the change:

$$\text{OR per 20 mm Hg increase in DBP} = e^{20 \times 0.01} = e^{0.2} = 1.22$$

Therefore, a 20 mm Hg increase in DBP is associated with 1.22-fold greater odds of stroke.

Determining what constitutes a clinically meaningful change in a continuous variable such as blood pressure can be difficult. One commonly used approach is to report the odds ratio per SD increase in a variable. For example, if the regression coefficient is 0.02, and the SD is 40, then the odds ratio per SD is:

$$\text{Odds ratio per SD increase} = e^{0.02 \times 40} = e^{0.8} = 2.2$$

Sometimes, a predictor variable is continuous but has a range that is <1.0. For example, if you are looking at a biochemical measurement that varies from 0 to 0.20 $\mu g/L$, it is extremely misleading to calculate the odds ratio from the regression coefficient for a "one-unit" change in that variable: It represents a change that is 5-fold bigger than the range of possible values. In this sort of situation, using the SD may be especially important. For example, if the regression coefficient was 8.0 and the SD was 0.04, then the odds ratio would be almost 3,000 for a biologically meaningless one-unit change but a much more reasonable odds ratio of 1.4 for a 1-SD change.

What if a variable reduces the risk of the outcome, such as aspirin use and stroke? Then the regression coefficient would be negative, and the odds ratio would be <1.0. For example, the regression coefficient for aspirin use might be −0.4. The odds ratio is:

$$\text{OR for use of aspirin} = e^{-0.4} = 0.7$$

Therefore, use of aspirin is associated with an odds ratio of 0.7 or a 30% decrease in the odds of stroke.

It is imperative that you verify how your variables were coded. If you think smokers are coded as 1 and nonsmokers as 0, and it is actually the other way around (or that smokers are coded as 1 and nonsmokers as 2), then you will completely misinterpret the meaning of the regression coefficient in the models.

What about confidence intervals? These are easy to estimate. The bounds of the confidence intervals extend 1.96 times the standard error above and below the point estimate.

Lower bound for the 95% confidence interval for the OR = $e^{b - 1.96 \times SE}$

Upper bound for the 95% confidence interval for the odds ratio = $e^{b + 1.96 \times SE}$

A very close approximation is:

Lower bound for the 95% confidence interval for the OR = $e^{b - 2 \times SE}$

Upper bound for the 95% confidence interval for the odds ratio = $e^{b + 2 \times SE}$

For example, if $b = 0.4$ and SE = 0.15, then:

$$OR = e^b = e^{0.4} = 1.5$$

Lower bound for the 95% confidence interval for OR = $e^{0.4 - 0.3} = e^{0.1} = 1.1$

Upper bound for the 95% confidence interval for OR = $e^{0.4 + 0.3} = e^{0.7} = 2.0$

As a check, make sure that the value for the lower confidence bound multiplied by the upper confidence bound equals the OR squared:

$$OR^2 = (\text{lower bound}) \times (\text{upper bound})$$

$$1.5^2 = 1.1 \times 2.0$$

For example, if OR is 2.0 and the lower confidence bound is 0.8, then the upper confidence bound should be 5.0 because $2^2 = 0.8 \times 5.0$.

6

Tables

A well-constructed table has just the right amount of information, presented in a format that makes its purpose clear at a glance. The simple format of a table—the facts, neatly lined up—is its chief strength. Compared with text, tables serve two main purposes: (1) they present facts more compactly and (2) they provide the possibility of side-by-side comparisons of those facts. In addition, perhaps because some investigators write poorly, many readers have developed the habit of ignoring or skimming the text of a results section while just looking at the tables.

This tendency has encouraged many authors to use tables for small but important packets of information. However, little bits of information can usually be presented more effectively in well-written text. Count the number of distinct pieces of information you plan to include in your table. If there are fewer than five or six, text will suffice. However, do not bulk up a table just to make it look more impressive—the excessive detail will detract from your overall message. For example, a table of the respiratory pathogens during the last several years at your hospital should list just the 10 or so most common isolates, with the others relegated to a footnote.

Once your manuscript is published, the reader's eyes will be attracted to the tables and figures because they look nice when printed in a journal. Tables and figures can, however, present substantial problems while your article is in manuscript form. Because they are appended after the text, reviewers must flip back and forth to look at them while they read your manuscript. Tables are also much less visually appealing in manuscript form, and a reviewer may wind up leafing through them after reading the text. Therefore, it is essential that you give total attention to the careful development of your text.

As mentioned in the previous chapter, a widespread practice among scientific writers is to prepare the tables and figures first and then write some brief text to string them together ("Table 1 shows…, Table 2 shows…, In Figure 1 it is shown…"). However, such a strategy guarantees that reviewers will spend less time reading your manuscript than it may merit. They will just look at the tables and figures. Instead, use text to introduce the tables and figures and to comment on what they show.

Some authors treat tables like parking lots—as convenient places to store large amounts of data. Although they may solve the "what in the world am I going to do with all these data" problem, sprawling tables can defeat readers who are looking for a particular piece of data. Clear signposts that label the rows and columns in a logical order will be needed.

If, like most junior investigators, you will be preparing your tables, spend some time learning how to use the table-making features of your word-processing or spreadsheet program. Alternatively, at least learn how to make columns or how to use the different tab key functions.

◆ TABLE COMPONENTS

All tables share several basic elements. These include a title; row and column headings; the rows themselves; the data; and footnotes (Table 6.1).

TABLE 6.1	A Descriptive Title, Such as "Structure of a Typical Table"[a]	
This Heading Describes the Rows	**This Heading Labels the First Column**	**This Heading Labels the Second Column**
What is in the first row (units)	DATA	DATA
What is in the second row (units)	DATA	DATA

[a]Not all tables follow this format.

The *title* should be sufficiently descriptive to tell the reader what will appear in the table. "Results of the Study" is not good enough. Imagine reproducing the table without any accompanying text. Does the title contain enough information about the study so that the table still makes sense? Many journals have specific rules about what needs to be in a title, such as the type and number of subjects or the time period of the study. However, do not burden the reader with a title that obscures the point in verbiage that describes your methodology in excruciating detail (Table 6.2). The rules on which words in a table title should be capitalized will vary from journal to journal. Look at the tables in the publication in which you are interested and style your table titles the same way.

TABLE 6.2	Poor Titles, with Better Alternatives
Poor Titles	**Better Titles**
Characteristics of subjects	Characteristics of the 154 subjects at the time of enrollment
Effects of treatment of hypertension	Comparison of diuretic therapy versus placebo among 283 patients with hypertension: 6-month results
Predictors of quality of life	Factors associated with quality of life among patients with cirrhosis: Multivariate models
Independent ($P < 0.05$) predictors of quality of life using logistic regression following step-wise selection procedures, using the criteria of reference 6	Factors associated with differences in quality of life among patients with cirrhosis: Multivariate models

The most important decision you will make about a table is one that many authors never think about, namely, what should form the rows and what should be the columns. The purpose of a table determines how you construct it: form follows function. *It is easier to compare two numbers (or even three) that are side by side than to compare numbers that are above and below each other.* If, for example, the purpose of the table is to show how a particular measurement changed over time, then the different times (baseline, week 1, and week 6) should be the column headings (Table 6.3). If the primary comparison is between groups (say, smokers, and nonsmokers), then those two groups should be the column headings.

TABLE 6.3	Selected Hemodynamic Measurements (Mean ± SD) at Baseline and during Follow-up, in 58 Subjects with Hypertension		
	Week of Treatment[a]		
Measurement	**Baseline**	**1**	**6**
Heart rate (per minute)	76 ± 12	68 ± 8	65 ± 7
Systolic blood pressure (mm Hg)	162 ± 21	142 ± 18	138 ± 14
Diastolic blood pressure (mm Hg)	96 ± 12	82 ± 10	80 ± 6

[a]All measures showed significant ($P < 0.01$) differences from baseline at weeks 1 and 6.

The first column of most data tables is simply a list of the variables that are presented in the table. The heading for that column should contain a simple description of what appears in each row, such as "Characteristics" or "Selected predictors." Sometimes this is obvious and the first column does not need a header. As much as possible, place the units for the variables in parentheses immediately after the row descriptions. The meaning of every item in a table should be obvious; the reader should not have to refer back to the text.

The *headings* for the other columns in the table should be informative. Avoid using terms such as *Group A, Group B, Group* C, and so on. Doing so makes readers constantly refer back to the text to remind themselves what *Group A* means. Instead, use a brief phrase that summarizes characteristics of Group A (e.g., cirrhotic, steroid-dependent), which can be described in greater detail in the text. Column headings, including the one that describes what will appear in the rows, should be easy to distinguish (e.g., bold or italicized). Some journals prefer that the size of the sample be included in the title, whereas others prefer that this information be listed under the appropriate column heading.

Keep footnotes to a minimum. They should be used only to explain essential details and abbreviations. A table that is cluttered with asterisks, tiny letters and numbers, and funny little symbols in a random order is a sure sign of someone who has allowed his or her word processor to run amok.

To determine how to sequence your footnotes, use this rule: By order of appearance in lines from top to bottom, within a line from left to right. To "number" your footnotes, use the following symbols, in this order: *, †, ‡, §, ||, and ¶. After you have used these six symbols, you use them again, doubled for the next six footnotes (e.g., **, ††, etc.), tripled for the next six, and so on. It can sometimes be tricky to find some of these symbols, other than the asterisk (which is shift-8, of course), in your word-processing program. Look in the Insert menu for the Symbols menu. The dagger (†) and double dagger (‡) may be found under General Punctuation; the Section sign (§) and Pilcrow or paragraph sign (¶) are found in Latin-1; and the double vertical line (||), which is actually two vertical lines repeated, is from the Latin alphabet. If you are going to use a lot of table footnotes, it may be worth creating keystroke shortcuts for these.

Capitalize the first letter of each line and column heading in your table (Table 6.4).

TABLE 6.4	Self-Reported Exercise in Smokers and Nonsmokers[a]	
Measurement of Exercise	**Smokers (*n* = 78)**	**Nonsmokers (*n* = 114)**
Times per week (mean ± SD, median)		
Any exercise	1 ± 2, 0	3 ± 2, 2
Exercise that causes sweat	0.5 ± 1, 0	2 ± 1, 1
Kcal per week (mean ± SD)	230 ± 110	460 ± 180
Blocks walked per week (mean, interquartile range)	20 (4, 56)	36 (12, 88)
Climb at least one flight of stairs daily (%)	25	48

[a]There were significant (*P* < 0.05) differences between smokers and nonsmokers in all variables.

Many journals present data in a slightly different way, illustrated in Table 6.5, using a subheader for the data columns that explains what the numbers represent. This avoids having to repeat mean ± SD or *N* (%) in the rows. To avoid ambiguity about the meaning of the data, present percentages within parentheses and standard deviations after plus–minus signs. Use the Insert Symbols menu for the plus–minus sign (±), rather than just underlining the plus sign.

TABLE 6.5	Self-Reported Exercise Habits of Smokers and Nonsmokers[a]	
Exercise Habit	**Smokers (*n* = 78)**	**Nonsmokers (*n* = 114)**
	N (%); or Mean ± SD, median; or Mean (interquartile range)	
Times per week		
Any exercise	1 ± 2, 0	3 ± 2, 2
Exercise that causes sweat	0.5 ± 1, 0	2 ± 1, 1
Kcal per week	230 ± 110	460 ± 180
Blocks walked per week	20 (4, 56)	36 (12, 88)
Climb at least one flight of stairs daily	19 (25)	55 (48)

[a]There were significant (*P* < 0.05) differences between smokers and nonsmokers in all variables.

Use your word-processing program to align the numbers in each column, either using the decimal or centering tab feature, or by centering the entries in the cells of the table layout. Leave enough space between the columns so that individual entries are distinct. If you do not have enough room to do this, turn the table 90° and use a horizontal format. Center the column headings over the columns.

Make sure that you cite all the tables in the text, almost always in the results section of your manuscript. Tables should be numbered in the order of citation.

Most journals do not require that you draw lines below the titles and above the footnotes, italicize the column headings, or use a different font (one without serifs, the short lines that angle off the ends of letters). However, these niceties do make tables neater for the reviewers. Similarly, although it is not absolutely essential to get the order of a table's footnotes correct in the first copy of the manuscript that you submit, following the rules demonstrates your attention to detail.

TYPES OF TABLES

When considering whether to include a particular table, you may find it useful to ask yourself what message that table is meant to convey. The purpose of the table will guide the table's format (Table 6.6).

TABLE 6.6	Common Types of Tables and the Messages They Might Convey
Lists (of facts, diagnoses, and criteria)	
The 10 most common mnemonics used by medical students	
Characteristics of subjects	
Clinical characteristic of patients with painless hematuria	
What happened to the subjects during the study?	
Outcomes during 6-year follow-up in 241 patients after first myocardial infarction	
Comparisons of groups of subjects	
Comparison of demographic characteristics of cases and control	
Predictors of what happened to the subjects	
Factors associated with falling asleep in grand rounds	
Results of a complicated multivariate analysis	
Independent predictors of mortality in a cohort of 834 factory workers	

There are other messages that are not very interesting, and they will not make very good tables. These sorts of tables should be included in a manuscript only if they absolutely have to be there, such as in a technical report (Table 6.7).

TABLE 6.7	Messages That Are Either Too Big or Too Dull for a Table
Mean and standard deviation for every variable measured in the study	
Differential diagnosis of fever	
Numbers of patients enrolled in each of 20 centers	
Sodium concentrations 1, 3, 6, and 9 months after diuretic therapy was started in all 39 subjects	

Tables of Lists

Some tables are just lists of items, such as diagnostic criteria or the types of bacteria that cause urinary tract infections. The essential decisions are what to include and in what order. A list may not have an intrinsic order, such as the causes of hyperkalemia, or it may have an order that is essential to the point you are trying to make, such as the frequency of symptoms in a patient with Cushing syndrome. Beware of imposing an order that confuses your point. It makes little sense, for example, to alphabetize urinary tract pathogens (Table 6.8).

TABLE 6.8	Common Urinary Tract Pathogens (Alphabetical)
Candida species	
Enterococcus species	
Escherichia coli	
Proteus mirabilis	
Staphylococcus aureus	

A better approach is to list the pathogens by frequency, perhaps subcategorized by type. A more informative titles and headings also help (Table 6.9).

Table 6.9 demonstrates an important rule: Avoid using percents of percents. Each percentage in a column should refer to the same denominator. If you want the reader to notice that half of the gram-positive species were *S. aureus*, then say so in the text: "We cultured different organisms (Table 6.9). *Staphylococcus aureus* accounted for half of the gram-positive culture results." Note that the percentages for the two most common types of gram-negative pathogens in the table do not sum to the total for all gram-negative bacteria; this immediately informs the reader that other species were seen. If these species matter, they could be included in a footnote. The percentages for specific gram-negative (and gram-positive) organisms are offset slightly to indicate that they are a part of the total for that group. The numbers of each pathogen have been omitted intentionally; they would be included only if you wanted readers to be able to check your arithmetic.

TABLE 6.9	Frequency of Pathogens in 840 Women with Lower Urinary Tract Infections	
Type of Pathogen		**Frequency (%)**
Gram-negative bacteria		63
Escherichia coli		55
Proteus mirabilis		4
Gram-positive bacteria		26
Staphylococcus aureus		13
Enterococcus species		9
Candida species		3
Other or no organism identified		8

Tables of Subject Characteristics

Usually, the first table in a manuscript orients the reader to the study participants. This table should include the essential characteristics of the subjects in your sample, such as age, sex, and race. Commonly, disease stage and selected risk factors are also important. Ask yourself what readers will want to know about the subjects. How does the example (Table 6.10) look?

TABLE 6.10	Characteristics of the Subjects[a]	
Male	594	(49.75%)
Female	600	(50.25%)
Age	64.47 ± 5.23	
History of diabetes	103	(8.63%)
History of CHD	56	(4.69%)
Body weight	74.1 ± 17.3	
Shoe size	9.2 ± 2.1	
Calories per month	62,125.4 ± 15,781.2	

[a]This is not a good table; see Table 6.11 for an improved version.

At first glance, the table may look fine. However, it is loaded with problems. The title is generic; it does not specify which subjects and how many. Stating the proportions of subjects who were male, and then doing the same for female subjects, is not necessary. The extraneous variables and unnecessary precision are distracting; will anyone really care about the subjects' mean shoe size, or that exactly 8.63% of subjects had a history of diabetes? The table mixes dichotomous data, such as history of diabetes, with continuous data such as body weight. There is an undefined abbreviation (CHD); the columns are not labeled; the units are not provided for age and body weight and they do not make sense for caloric intake; and the meaning of the plus–minus values is not specified. Consider the improved version, Table 6.11.

TABLE 6.11	Characteristics of the 1,194 Subjects Enrolled in the Better Eating Trial
Characteristics	**N (%) or Mean ± SD**
Male	594 (50)
History of diabetes	103 (9)
History of coronary heart disease	56 (5)
Age (year)	64 ± 5
Body weight (kg)	74 ± 17
Calories/per day	2, 070 ± 530

The text that accompanies the table might simply read, "There were similar numbers of men and women in the study (Table 6.11); 33% of the subjects were over 65 years of age, and 25% were more than 10 kg above ideal body weight. Most were free of chronic medical problems."

Occasionally, it is worthwhile to divide (stratify) the information on the subjects into two groups (e.g., men and women). This type of table is most useful if there are important differences between the two groups, which should be pointed out in the accompanying text: "Diabetes was 40% more common among women, whereas male subjects were more than twice as likely to have reported a history of heart disease." The text can also be used to emphasize other aspects of the sample, such as the fact that the numbers of men and women were similar or that the overall mean age was 64 years (Table 6.12).

TABLE 6.12	Characteristics of the 1,194 Subjects Enrolled in the Better Eating Trial, by Sex	
	Men (*n* = 594)	Women (*n* = 600)
	n (%) or Mean ± SD	
Age (years)	62 ± 5	66 ± 6
Body weight (kg)	80 ± 16	68 ± 18
History of diabetes	40 (7)	63 (10)
History of coronary heart disease	38 (7)	18 (3)

If the manuscript reports the results of a randomized trial, then the characteristics of the subjects need to be presented for each of the study groups. Percentages rather than numbers of subjects may be easier to follow. This is especially true if the numbers of subjects in the groups vary substantially (e.g., because twice as many subjects were randomly assigned to the treatment as to the control group). Traditionally, *P* values comparing the groups are also provided to demonstrate the adequacy of randomization (Table 6.13).

TABLE 6.13	Characteristics of the 1,194 Subjects Enrolled in the Better Eating Trial, by Randomization Status		
	Special Diet (*n* = 797)	Control (*n* = 397)	*P*
	n (%) or Mean ± SD		
Age (years)	64.8 ± 5.4	65.1 ± 5.8	0.38
Body weight (kg)	74 ± 16	73 ± 16	0.32
History of diabetes	65 (8)	38 (10)	0.51
History of coronary heart disease	40 (5)	16 (4)	0.38

Tables That Tell What Happened

In some types of studies, such as cohort studies and clinical trials that follow a group of subjects for a particular period, it is necessary to tell the reader what occurred during the study. If you are only interested in one or two outcomes, then text will suffice: "Of the 682 subjects, 116 (17%) died during the study." Tables are useful if there are several outcomes of interest (e.g., death, myocardial infarction, and hospitalization). Tables are also valuable when you wish to categorize outcomes into different classes, such as deaths owing to cancer and deaths owing to cardiovascular disease—especially if you want to subcategorize them further, such as by types of cancer.

Tables that tell what happened can quickly become filled with superfluous detail. For example, if you present the number of fatal myocardial infarctions and strokes and the total number of deaths owing to cardiovascular disease, you need not present the number of other cardiovascular deaths. Again, the percentages should all refer to the same denominator (all deaths). If you want to indicate what proportion of cardiovascular deaths resulted from strokes, do so in text: "Stroke was responsible for 28% of the deaths owing to cardiovascular diseases" (Table 6.14).

TABLE 6.14	Mortality during 3.5 Years of Follow-Up in 682 Participants
Cause of Death	**Number (%)**
Cardiovascular disease	60 (8.8)
Myocardial infarction	34 (5.0)
Anterior	18 (2.6)
Inferior	12 (1.8)
Stroke	17 (2.5)
Cancer	41 (6.0)
Lung	12 (1.8)
Colon	10 (1.5)
Breast	9 (1)
Others	15 (2.2)
Total	116 (17.0)

There is another way to present the same data, this time emphasizing the proportions of death from each cause, rather than the absolute risk of each cause (Table 6.15). In this table, it is somewhat easier to see that cardiovascular diseases caused about half of the deaths and cancer about one-third.

TABLE 6.15	Causes of 116 Deaths during 3.5 Years of Follow-Up in 682 Participants
Cause of Death	**N (% of All Deaths)**
Cardiovascular disease	60 (52)
Myocardial infarction	34 (29)
Anterior	18 (17)
Inferior	12 (12)
Stroke	17 (15)
Cancer	41 (35)
Lung	12 (10)
Colon	10 (9)
Breast	9 (8)
Others	15 (13)

Tables That Compare Groups

When you are presenting comparisons of two or more groups, you are presenting two types of information: the measurements themselves in each of the groups and the differences between the groups. You must decide which of those two types of information is more important because that will influence how you organize the table.

Consider Table 6.16 that compares the characteristics of patients with asthma and those with chronic obstructive pulmonary disease in a study of the effects of intensive vacuuming of the subjects' carpets. Here the emphasis is on the characteristics, rather than on the differences between the two types of patients. Everyone already knows that the two types of patients are very different. A simple indication that there were statistically significant differences is all that is needed.

TABLE 6.16	Characteristics (Mean ± SD) of the 117 Subjects Enrolled in the Vacuum Away Dust Study, by Type of Pulmonary Disease		
Characteristics (Unit)	**Asthma (n = 51)**	**COPD[a] (n = 66)**	**P**
Age (years)	32 ± 8	66 ± 6	<0.001
Forced expiratory volume, 1 second (L)	2.5 ± 0.6	1.2 ± 0.8	<0.001
Peak expiratory flow (L/minute)	320 ± 110	230 ± 90	<0.001
Prednisone dose (mg/day)	15 ± 20	12 ± 18	>0.25

[a]COPD, chronic obstructive pulmonary disease. (This is an abbreviation that is actually helpful because it is widely recognized and unambiguous.)

When the emphasis is on the comparison—as in a randomized trial comparing a drug and a placebo, or in a study to determine the predictors of response to vacuuming—more is required. The reader will not only want to know whether there is a statistically significant difference but the size of that difference as well. In this case, the table must include a measure of that effect size and an estimate of how precisely the effect size was measured (its confidence interval; Table 6.17).

TABLE 6.17	Effect of Intensive Vacuuming on Pulmonary Function at 6 Months in the Vacuum Away Dust Study			
Measurement (Unit)	**Vacuum (n = 60)**	**Control (n = 57)**	**Vacuum–Control Difference (95% Confidence Interval)**	**P**
	Mean ± SD			
Forced expiratory volume, 1 second (L)	2.0 ± 0.6	1.6 ± 0.8	0.4 (0.1, 0.7)	<0.01
Peak expiratory flow (L/minute)	290 ± 80	260 ± 120	30 (5, 55)	<0.02
Prednisone dose (mg/day)	14 ± 12	10 ± 15	4 (−2, 6)	>0.15

Comparing an intervention group and a control group works fine for a randomized trial, but problems arise when you apply the same idea to a case–control or cohort study to compare cases that developed the outcome with those who did not (Table 6.18).

TABLE 6.18	Characteristics of the 1,346 Subjects, by Outcome[a]	
Characteristic (Unit)	Stroke (n = 122)	Controls (n = 1,224)
Mean ± SD age (years)	72 ± 5	66 ± 6
History of diabetes	40 (33%)	63 (5%)
Previous MI		
None	70 (57%)	1,103 (90%)
1	32 (26%)	105 (9%)
2	20 (16%)	16 (1%)

[a]This is not a good table; see Table 6.19 for an improved version.

Table 6.18 may look great, but it is terribly misleading. The reader will have to work hard to realize that the table does not indicate that 33% of the subjects with a history of diabetes developed strokes during the study; rather, 33% of those with strokes had diabetes. It is even harder to grasp the relation between stroke and the number of previous myocardial infarctions. The table fails to present what the reader wants to know: namely, whether the number of previous myocardial infarctions affects the incidence of stroke. Table 6.19 does a better job.

TABLE 6.19	Incidence of Stroke by Selected Characteristics of the 1,346 Subjects		
	Incidence of Stroke		
Characteristic	In Those with Characteristic	In Those without Characteristic	Relative Risk (95% Confidence Interval)
Age ≥70 years	12% (80/660)	6% (42/686)	2.0 (1.2–3.2)
Diabetes	39% (40/103)	7% (82/1,243)	5.8 (2.2–16)
Previous myocardial infarction	30% (52/173)	6% (70/1,173)	5.0 (3.2–8.0)

Putting the numbers in parentheses keeps the reader from being distracted from the purpose of the table, which is to demonstrate the incidence of stroke according to selected characteristics. The extremely high rate of stroke in subjects with two or more prior myocardial infarctions can be disclosed in the text: "The risk of stroke was 56% (20/36) among those subjects with two or more previous myocardial infarctions." Age—measured as a continuous variable—must be categorized for this sort of table. If you want to provide the mean ages of those with strokes and the controls, then do so in the text: "Those who had strokes were 6 years older than controls (72 ± 5 vs. 66 ± 6 years [mean ± SD], $P = 0.01$)."

Tables that are intended to show more complicated effects—such as the effects of smoking in men and in women—should use column subheaders for these subgroup or "nested" comparisons. The nested comparison should be the one that is *more* important, because the data in the table will be displayed side by side and will therefore be easier to compare. Table 6.20, for example, emphasizes the differences between smokers and nonsmokers: Smokers weigh less and have higher hemoglobin levels and leukocyte counts. This is true for both men and women.

TABLE 6.20	Association between Smoking Status and Selected Characteristics (Mean ± SD) in Men and Women between the Ages of 20 and 39 Years[a]			
	Men		Women	
Measurement	Smokers (n = 51)	Nonsmokers (n = 62)	Smokers (n = 33)	Nonsmokers (n = 35)
Weight (kg)	68 ± 8	72 ± 9	55 ± 6	66 ± 7
Hemoglobin (g/dL)	14.5 ± 2.0	13.3 ± 1.6	12.2 ± 1.8	11.3 ± 1.5
Leukocytes (1,000 per μL)	10.3 ± 2.4	9.1 ± 1.4	10.9 ± 2.1	9.2 ± 1.7

[a]All differences between smokers and nonsmokers are significant at $P < 0.05$.

Reversing the nesting process yields a table with the same information but in a much less accessible format. Although Table 6.21 shows that men are heavier—and have greater hemoglobin concentrations—than women, the effects of smoking are obscured.

TABLE 6.21	Effects of Sex on Selected Characteristics (Mean ± SD) of Smokers and Nonsmokers between the Ages of 20 and 39 Years[a]			
	Smokers		Nonsmokers	
Measurement	Men (n = 51)	Women (n = 33)	Men (n = 33)	Women (n = 35)
Weight (kg)	68 ± 8	55 ± 6	72 ± 9	66 ± 7
Hemoglobin (g/dL)	14.5 ± 2.0	12.2 ± 1.8	13.3 ± 1.6	11.3 ± 1.5
Leukocytes (1,000 per μL)	10.3 ± 2.4	10.9 ± 2.1	9.1 ± 1.4	9.2 ± 1.7

[a]All differences between smokers and nonsmokers are significant at $P < 0.05$. Note how difficult it is to compare the values in smokers with those in nonsmokers in this table, especially by comparison with Table 6.20.

Ordinarily, column headings are "bottom-justified." In other words, they should all align along the same bottom line (as in most of the tables in this section) just above the first row of data. However, if you have a nested table, as in the previous example, then the key column headings should be aligned along the same top line, or "top-justified."

Neither Table 6.20 nor Table 6.21 highlights another important result, namely, that the effects of smoking status on body weight are greater in women (smokers weigh 11 kg less than nonsmokers) than in men (a difference of 4 kg). In this case, because this is the only sex-specific difference, it will suffice to mention it in text. If there are several such differences, then two more columns should be added to the table and labeled as the difference between smokers and nonsmokers for both men and women. However, if these differences, or lack thereof, are very important—for example, if your research question addresses them—then a separate table of the sex-specific differences, with confidence intervals, should be included (Table 6.22).

TABLE 6.22	**Differences in the Effects of Smoking on Selected Characteristics in Men and Women between the Ages of 20 and 39 Years as Mean (95% Confidence Interval) Difference between Smokers and Nonsmokers**	
Measurement	**Men ($n = 113$)[a]**	**Women ($n = 68$)[a]**
Weight (kg)	4 (2–6)	11 (7–15)
Hemoglobin (g/dL)	1.2 (0.8–1.6)	0.9 (0.1–1.7)
Leukocytes (1,000 per μL)	1.2 (0.6–1.8)	1.7 (0.9–2.5)

[a]There were 51 men and 33 women who smoked. The effects of smoking are significantly different ($P < 0.05$) in men and women.

Tables with Many Rows and Columns

In some circumstances, there may not be a "control" group, so there is no "control column." Instead, a final column of averages should be included. Similarly, a final row of averages may also be useful (Table 6.23).

TABLE 6.23	**Choice of Postgraduate Training among 1,567 Fourth-Year Medical Students, by Selected Characteristics**						
Characteristic	**Medicine ($n = 219$)**	**Psychiatry ($n = 407$)**	**Pediatrics ($n = 125$)**	**Surgery ($n = 220$)**	**FP[a] ($n = 470$)**	**Others[a] ($n = 126$)**	**Total**
Women, %	10	40	54	45	38	23	46
Nonwhite, %	8	12	6	11	18	5	12
Varsity athlete, %	24	4	2	3	3	5	4
History of psychotherapy, %	8	12	63	23	32	9	28
Total choosing discipline, %	14	26	8	14	30	8	100

[a]FP, family practice.

Table 6.23 is challenging, but with a little effort one can determine what percentage of fourth-year students were women (46%), what percentage elected each of the possible training choices (8% chose pediatrics), and the differences by type of training program. The table does not tell you the percentage of women who chose psychiatry training programs; if that information was of primary interest, the rows and columns should have been reversed.

It is difficult to present effect sizes when comparing three or more groups. With three groups (A, B, and C), there are three comparisons (A vs. B, A vs. C, and B vs. C). Including three columns of effect sizes with confidence intervals makes for a cluttered table (with 6 groups, there are 15 effect sizes). This problem often manifests when you are comparing several doses of a drug. One tempting option is to select the "biggest effect." This is seldom the best choice, unless the investigators specify in advance the dose they believe will be both safe and efficacious.

Another option combines two of the groups (low dose and high dose) and compares them with the placebo. If there are just a few statistically significant between-dose differences, they can be highlighted in the text. Another choice, if there is a dose–response relationship, presents the results as a figure that makes the effect sizes obvious. A final option involves having another table that just shows the differences between the groups. Do not make the mistake of not presenting the effect sizes at all.

Some authors prefer to develop some sort of system using asterisks and daggers, or lowercase letters, to indicate the differences that are statistically significant and those that are not. If you do this, do not get carried away. Decide on the comparisons and levels of statistical significance that really matter and provide the *P* values only for those comparisons. Remember that before you do pairwise comparisons, you need to demonstrate that there is a statistically significant difference across all the groups (see the discussion of analysis of variance [ANOVA] in Chapter 5 for more on this problem).

Tables of Multivariable Results

As elaborate statistical techniques for data analysis have become more available, investigators are faced with the difficult problem of figuring out how to present the results of those analyses in an accessible manner. Regression models yield all sorts of factors—regression coefficients, standard errors, slopes, partial correlation coefficients, and *P* values among them. The primary task is to present the effect of the predictor variable (e.g., cystatin C level) on the outcome of interest (e.g., coronary heart disease) in a clinically meaningful way. For a dichotomous outcome, this usually involves presenting how a clinically meaningful change in the predictor variable changes the risk of that outcome. The 95% confidence interval for that change should also be provided.

Why is Table 6.24 almost completely unintelligible? First, most readers will have no idea of the meaning of regression coefficients or standard errors. Second, even if they do understand these statistical concepts, they will not know the units of change in the predictor. Does the regression coefficient for sex refer to the difference between men and women, or between women and men? Does the coefficient for age refer to the change per year, per 10 years, or comparing older and younger subjects? To what does smoking refer?

A simple fix involves using clinically meaningful terms, such as the odds ratios, and providing units for each of the predictor variables. On occasion, the units will be implicit, such as that men were compared with women. More often, the units

TABLE 6.24	Independent Predictors of Coronary Heart Disease among 2,124 Middle-Aged Subjects, Using Logistic Regression Models[a]		
Predictor	**Regression Coefficient**	**Standard Error**	**P**
Sex	0.51	0.22	0.01
Age	0.05	0.01	<0.0001
Serum cholesterol	0.3	0.15	0.05
Systolic blood pressure	0.7	0.3	0.02
Smoking	1.1	0.3	<0.0001

[a]This is not a good table; Table 6.25 is much better.

need to be provided to indicate that, for example, current smokers were compared with people who never smoked, rather than current nonsmokers (Table 6.25). If you do not know how to convert logistic regression coefficients into clinically meaningful terms, see the Appendix to Chapter 5.

TABLE 6.25	Independent Predictors of Coronary Heart Disease among 2,124 Middle-Aged Subjects		
Predictor	**Relative Risk[a]**	**95% Confidence Interval**	**P**
Male	1.7	1.1–2.6	0.01
Age (per 10 years)	1.6	1.4–2.0	<0.0001
Serum cholesterol (per 20 mg/dL)	1.3	1.0–1.8	0.05
Systolic blood pressure (per 10 mm Hg)	2.0	1.1–3.6	0.02
Current smoker (vs. never smoked)	3.0	1.7–5.4	<0.0001

[a]Relative risks approximated with odds ratios from a logistic regression model.

However, even the solution proposed by Table 6.25 is not perfect because it fails to convey a key point—that the risk of coronary heart disease is much greater in those with multiple risk factors. A figure (see the next chapter) might make that obvious.

Sometimes it is worth presenting a table that indicates to the reader the variables that were associated with the outcome in univariate models but not in multivariate models, and why. For example, thinness may have been associated with the subsequent development of lung cancer in a univariate model, but it may no longer be associated in a model that accounts for cigarette smoking because persons who smoke tend to be thin (Table 6.26).

TABLE 6.26	Univariate Predictors That Were No Longer Associated with Lung Cancer after Adjustment for Other Factors in Multivariate Models		
Predictor	**Univariate Relative Risk (95% CI)[a]**	**Multivariate Relative Risk (95% CI)**	**Removed By**
Thinness (<90% IBW)	2.1 (1.3–3.1)	1.4 (0.8–2.5)	Subject's smoking
Income (per $10,000)	0.8 (0.6–1.0)	1.0 (0.8–1.2)	Age
Spouse's smoking (yes/no)	3.1 (1.5–6.2)	1.3 (0.7–2.2)	Subject's smoking
Body weight (per 5 kg)	0.6 (0.4–0.8)	0.9 (0.7–1.2)	Disease stage

[a]Relative risks approximated with odds ratios.
IBW, ideal body weight; CI, confidence interval.

 ## WHEN TO COMBINE TABLES

Consider combining tables that have the same or similar column headings. Not only does this save space, but juxtaposing data often suggest new ways of looking at your results. See, for example, Tables 6.27 and 6.28.

| TABLE 6.27 | Results of Treatment of Migraine with Sumatran Tea | | | |

Outcome	Tea Group (%)	Control Group (%)	Tea–Control Difference (%)	95% Confidence Interval
Headache	64	79	−15	(−8% to −22%)
Nausea	35	38	−3	(3% to −9%)
Photophobia	19	21	−2	(6% to −10%)
Any of these symptoms	70	82	−12	(−4% to −20%)

Note the use of the word "to" (6% to −10%), rather than a dash (6% − −10%), to avoid confusion with the minus sign.

| TABLE 6.28 | Side Effects of Treatment of Migraine with Sumatran Tea | | | |

Side Effect	Tea Group (%)	Control Group (%)	Tea–Control Difference (%)	95% Confidence Interval
Diarrhea	26	9	17	(12% to 22%)
Reflux esophagitis	15	12	3	(−3% to 9%)
Abdominal cramps	11	9	2	(−6% to 10%)
Any side effects	32	23	9	(4% to 14%)

Combining the two tables (Table 6.29) makes it clear that the side effects of treatment are of a magnitude and severity commensurate with its benefits, an observation that was less obvious when there were two tables. Combining tables of benefits and side effects would not make sense, however, if the side effects of a therapy, such as nausea or skin rash, were not commensurate with its benefits, such as reduced cancer deaths.

| TABLE 6.29 | Results and Side Effects of Treatment of Migraine with Sumatran Tea | | | |

Outcome	Tea Group (%)	Control Group (%)	Tea–Control Difference (%)	95% Confidence Interval
Headache	64	79	−15	(−8% to −22%)
Nausea	35	38	−3	(3% to −9%)
Photophobia	19	21	−2	(6% to −10%)
Diarrhea	26	9	17	(12% to 22%)
Reflux esophagitis	15	12	3	(−3% to 9%)
Abdominal cramps	11	9	2	(−6% to 10%)
Free of all symptoms or side effects	88	87	1	(5% to −3%)

WHAT SHOULD BE LEFT OUT OF A TABLE?

Mega tables of everything that you have measured are not useful. Indeed, they may be counterproductive, if the important or significant differences that you have found are ascribed to multiple hypothesis testing ("Look at how many different things they compared."). But, do not just include measurements that were statistically significant; this is simply dishonest.

The best prevention against accusations of multiple hypothesis testing is to have a few prespecified hypotheses and to indicate which ones they are. If you happen to find fascinating but unanticipated results, these can be included with a clear notation that they were unexpected ("We were surprised to find that...") to emphasize that the results may have occurred by chance and need to be confirmed.

PREPARING THE TABLE IN YOUR MANUSCRIPT

Unless it is absolutely unavoidable, do your best to limit each table to a single page. Your reviewers will thank you. You can always provide a double-spaced, 12-point, three-page version for a journal's technical editor after the article is accepted. If you must, turn the table so that it prints in a horizontal or landscape format (use the Page Setup command). The single-page rule holds even if you must use a slightly smaller font and cannot double-space; a 10-point font and 1.5-line spacing will suffice. You can use the Page Setup command to reduce the size of the page to, say, 80%. However, do not singlespace or use a microscopic font.

As you finish each table, ask the questions in the Checklist for Tables at the end of this chapter.

A FINAL TEST

Look at Table 6.30 that compares pediatric patients less than 2 years old undergoing surgery for congenital abnormalities at two university hospitals (Group I) and three community hospitals (Group II). Now, ask yourself, how can this table be made easier to follow and more informative?

TABLE 6.30	Comparison of Selected Characteristics of the Two Groups of Subjects		
Characteristic	**Group I**	**Group II**	**P**
Male	74/112 = 66%	33/68 = 49%	a
Female	28/112 = 34%	35/68 = 51%	a
CHD	77/112 = 69%	50/68 = 74%	NS
Cost in dollars	$29,323 ± $13,358	$31,482 ± 16,552	NS
Age (years)	0.5 ± 0.5	0.6 ± 0.4	NS
Premature	92/112 = 82%	43/68 = 63%	a
<32 weeks	47%	41%	NS
<28 weeks	18%	3%	a

[a] $P < 0.05$. NS, nonsignificant.

Table 6.31 illustrates one way of improving the table. How does this compare with the improved version you came up with?

TABLE 6.31	Comparison of Characteristics of 180 Children Less Than 2 Years Old Undergoing Surgery for Congenital Abnormalities, at Two University Hospitals and Three Community Hospitals[a]		
Characteristics	**University Hospitals** (*n* = 112)	**Community Hospitals** (*n* = 68)	**P**
	N (%) or Mean ± SD		
Male	74 (66)	33 (49)	0.03
Congenital heart disease	77 (69)	50 (74)	>0.15
Premature birth (<38 weeks)	92 (82)	43 (63)	<0.01
28–32 weeks	32 (29)	26 (38)	>0.15
<28 weeks	20 (18)	2 (3)	<0.01
Age (months)	6.3 ± 6.1	7.2 ± 4.6	>0.15
Hospital charges (in $1,000)	29.3 ± 13.4	31.5 ± 16.6	>0.15

✔ CHECKLIST FOR

TABLES

1. Is the title sufficiently descriptive without being Tolstoy-esque?

2. Do the rows and columns line up neatly? Is each column centered under its heading? Are there denominators for the column headings? Are the headings boldfaced or italicized? Do the row characteristics have units?

3. Are there any unneeded data, repeated *N*s, excessive precision, or ambiguous abbreviations? Ask yourself: "Do I need it? Do I need it in such glorious detail? Do I need to abbreviate it?"

4. Is the meaning of every item obvious without referring to the text?

5. Are all the tables cited in the text? Are they cited in order?

6. After you have completed all your tables, ask if two or more of them can be combined.

7

Figures

Most manuscripts include figures, perhaps because the adage that "one picture is worth a thousand words" strikes most authors as true. However, many published figures turn out to have been worth only 10 or 20 words. Because preparing and modifying figures takes much more time than writing and revising a couple of sentences, make sure you actually need a figure before you start preparing it. In addition, although figures are terrific at displaying overall effects, they are usually poor at conveying specific measurements. If the details matter, use a table instead, or supplement the figure with the exact values in the text.

There are three common types of figures in clinical articles: photographs, diagrams, and data presentations. A few general rules apply to the preparation of all three types. First, determine the figure's purpose. Then prepare—in pencil—several mock versions of the figure until you find one that demonstrates your point unambiguously. A confusing figure is much worse than no figure at all. If a reader has to spend 5 minutes getting oriented to your figure, you have not succeeded. A poorly photographed skin rash, a schema of the entire immune system, or a line graph that resembles a map of the New York City subway system will not be a useful addition to your manuscript.

Look through the examples in the chapter for a "model figure" that seems to fit the type of results you wish to present. All of the figures in the chapter can be made using standard spreadsheet software; none of them will take more than a half hour to prepare for a reasonably experienced user of the software.

At the same time, begin thinking about the *legend* for the figure, which describes the purpose and contents of that figure. Not being able to develop a suitable legend is often an early clue that the figure may not achieve its purpose. If you find yourself having to prepare a convoluted three-sentence legend, you may need to reconsider the figure.

Usually a figure can show only a few results. If you are planning to demonstrate several results, consider having more than one figure or moving some data from the figure to a table or to the text. An extremely complicated figure, such as, "Everything known about homocysteine metabolism," although it may appear to be a useful summary, tends to overwhelm the reader with so much detail that the essential points are lost. While such a figure might be useful in a review article, it would rarely belong in a manuscript presenting original data.

When you have completed your figure mockups, show them to a few colleagues who have not worked on the manuscript. Provide the legends but no other explanation and ask whether each figure's main point is clear. If it is not, redo the pencil versions of the mockups. Doing this *before* you start to prepare the "real" figures will save you a lot of time in the long run.

PHOTOGRAPHS AS FIGURES

Photographs used as figures include gels, micrographs, radiographs, and pictures of patients. With a few exceptions, such as the heart shadow on a chest radiograph or erythrocytes in a blood smear, never assume that readers will recognize anything in a photograph. Label everything that is relevant, using arrows and arrowheads, asterisks, and commonly understood abbreviations (e.g., *WBC* for *white blood cell*). But even common abbreviations need to be defined in the figure's legend. If there are too many objects to point out, or if the items are difficult to distinguish, consider adding an explanatory cartoon with a schematic portrayal of the relevant structures and placing it alongside the photograph.

Photographs are relatively expensive to publish. Therefore, they should be used sparingly to make essential points. There is rarely a need to include yet another photograph of the butterfly rash of lupus, a chest radiograph showing pneumonia, or a photomicrograph showing small-vessel vasculitis.

A good way of checking the clarity of a photograph is to photocopy it. Is its main point still evident? If it is not, and you cannot produce a better photograph, include a neighboring cartoon (a hand-drawn rendering of the key features, labeled). Keep in mind that the better your article, the more likely future readers may be looking at a copy of a copy (of a copy ...) of the original.

Unless the scale of the photograph is obvious, include a ruler. Alternatively, indicate the magnification or reduction in the figure legend.

DIAGRAMS OR CARTOONS AS FIGURES

Appropriate subjects for depiction as a cartoon or diagram include interactions among molecules (such as the Krebs cycle), the flow of subjects in a study, the key details of a photograph, and genetic pedigrees. You should seriously consider getting professional assistance with these types of figures. Most desktop graphing and database programs do a reasonably good job of making graphic figures, but the same is not true for drawings. The boxes, arrows, and font are usually the wrong size, and subtle variations in the way you arrange items may give the figure an amateurish look when published. The results rarely look as good as a drawing done by a professional.

When in doubt, err on the side of simplicity rather than thoroughness. If no one can understand the purpose of the figure, its completeness will not be an asset. If you feel compelled to burden a figure with extraneous details, use a smaller font for the less important items.

Take advantage of a figure's ability to make interesting—or at least tolerable— what might otherwise be dull. For example, flow diagrams are useful for explaining complicated sampling schemes, algorithms, or protocols, especially if you include the numbers of subjects at each stage. As a general rule, sampling schemes are portrayed vertically (Fig. 7-1), whereas measurement algorithms are presented on a horizontal time axis (Fig. 7-2). Note that in Figure 7-1, boxes are used to distinguish subjects who are no longer enrolled in the study; those who remain at each stage are included in ovals.

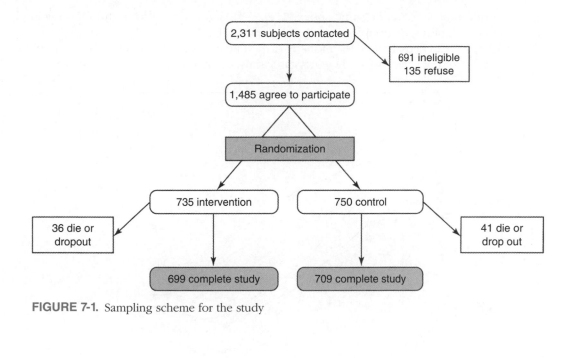

FIGURE 7-1. Sampling scheme for the study

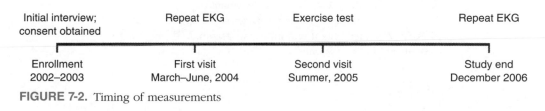

FIGURE 7-2. Timing of measurements

FIGURES THAT PRESENT NUMERICAL DATA

Figures that present numerical data offer the maximum difficulties. Because a graphical display of information, when done well, can be very effective, many authors try too hard to use a figure to convey their main results. Numerical figures should be used when the overall pattern is more important than the actual values. Always ask yourself, "Do I really need the figure? Does it make my point?"

Figures should have a minimum of four data points. A figure that shows that the rate of colon cancer is higher in men than in women or that diabetes is more common in Hispanics than in whites or blacks, is not worth making. Use text instead. The four-data-point minimum, however, does not apply to oral presentations, in which simple figures that convey limited amounts of data are appropriate. An audience can only incorporate a few pieces of information at a time.

The maximum amount of data depends on the type of figure. Unless the message you are trying to convey is that there is chaos in the data, having too many bars or lines or points will be counterproductive. Certain types of data are difficult to demonstrate in text or in tables, such as the values of a variable measured on several occasions in the same subject. A figure allows you to connect data points measured at different times in the same subject (Fig. 7-3). Figures are also useful for showing effects in different groups or at different times (Fig. 7-4).

Always check figures for mishaps or potential misunderstandings. For example, beware of lines that cross. They inevitably draw attention to the intersection, whether

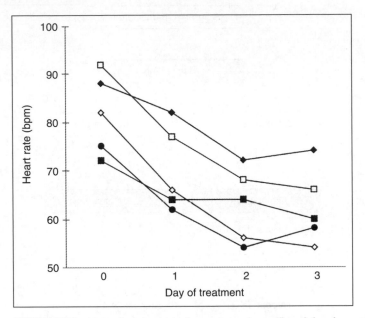

FIGURE 7-3. Mean heart rate in beats per minute (bpm) by day of treatment in five patients

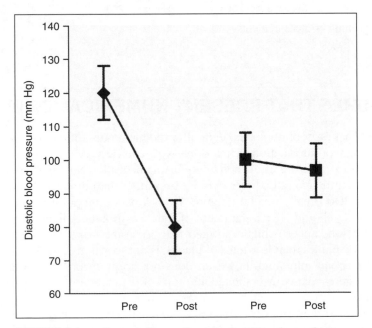

FIGURE 7-4. Differing effects of treatment with successol in patients with low renin (diamonds) and high renin (squares) hypertension. The filled shapes indicate the means; the bars indicate the 95% confidence intervals

it matters or not. In Figure 7-5, the reader's eye is drawn to what might have happened between Days 3 and 4, although it is just a coincidence that the lines cross at that time. Consider redrawing the figure using different scales to avoid the problem (Fig. 7-6).

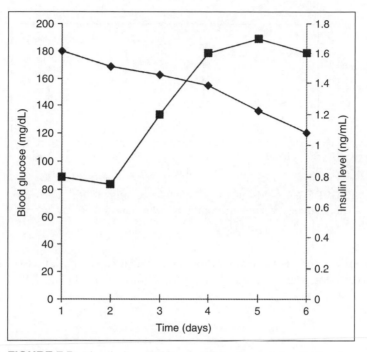

FIGURE 7-5. Blood glucose (diamonds) and serum insulin level (squares) versus time

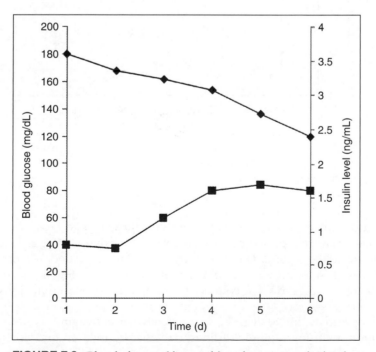

FIGURE 7-6. Blood glucose (diamonds) and serum insulin level (squares) versus time

Make sure the scale is right. Some measures, such as the confidence interval for an odds ratio, are not symmetric in linear scales. For example, a 95% confidence interval for an odds ratio of 2 might be from 1.1 to 3.6 (Fig. 7-7). Because

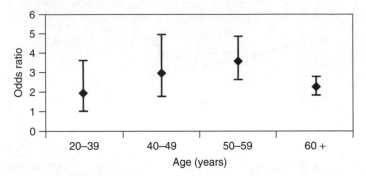

FIGURE 7-7. Odds ratio (95% confidence interval) for pancreatic cancer in heavy smokers compared with nonsmokers, by age

confidence intervals for odds ratios (and similar measures of association) are symmetric in a log scale, a logarithmic axis should be used (Fig. 7-8).

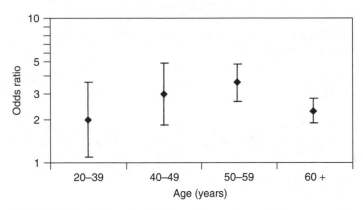

FIGURE 7-8. Odds ratio (95% confidence interval) for pancreatic cancer in heavy smokers compared with nonsmokers, by age (y axis on logarithmic scale)

Occasionally, it may not make sense for the y axis to cross the x axis at 0, or the scale may change for one of the axes. For example, the x axis may change from *days* at the beginning of the study to *months* at the end. If there is any potential for confusion, provide an explanation in the figure legend. If there is a break in one of the axes, do not connect points that lie on different sides of the break (Fig. 7-9).

Surprisingly, figures can be very effective at conveying the absence of an association, by using a tangle of lines, bars that bounce up and down, or dots that

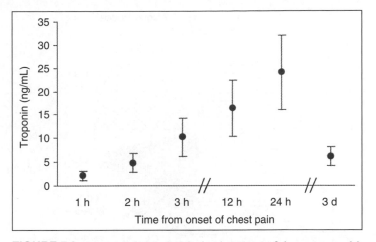

FIGURE 7-9. Mean troponin levels (with 95% confidence intervals) by time in patients with chest pain. Note that the time axis is not uniform

are scattered randomly (Fig. 7-10). Emphasize the absence of association in the legend and text so that readers arc not confused by your reason for including the figure.

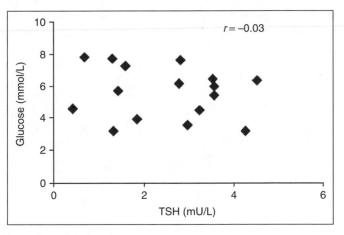

FIGURE 7-10. Lack of association between thyroid-stimulating hormone (TSH) and glucose levels in patients attending a weight-loss clinic

Types of Numerical Figures

The main types of numerical figures are pie charts, scatter plots, bar graphs, and line graphs. Pie charts should be avoided in written manuscripts. They are excellent for stories about baked goods, but they rarely have a place in clinical articles. They often do not look very professional (Fig. 7-11); more important, the data they contain can almost always be better presented in other forms, such as text if there are only a few slices in the pie or as a table if there are more.

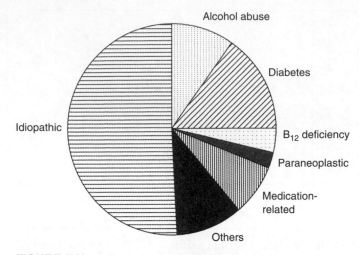

FIGURE 7-11. Causes of neuropathy in a sample of 112 primary care patients

Scatter plots can easily show the correlation, or lack of correlation, between two variables. A scatter plot of weight versus height (Fig. 7-12), for example, conveys the strong association between those variables effectively. Nearly all spreadsheet programs can easily make scatter plots and calculate regression coefficients (and sometimes even P values). You can "transform" data to plot the logarithm of one (or both) of the values or include the estimated regression line in the figure.

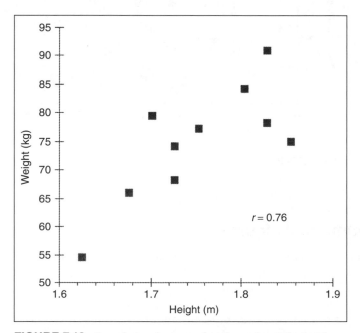

FIGURE 7-12. Correlation between height and weight in 10 subjects

Bar Graphs

Bar graphs are valuable for displaying results by categories of subjects, such as men and women, or for depicting conditions before and after an intervention. Bar graphs are most useful when what matters is the value of an outcome variable, rather than its confidence interval. Confidence intervals can be added (usually just the upper confidence limit) to a bar graph, but the figure will be more crowded and somewhat less elegant. If portraying the confidence interval is critical, consider using a line graph, with the mean shown by a dot or square and the confidence interval shown with lines (as in Fig. 7-4).

The key question in making a bar graph is how best to show the pattern of the data. Usually, that means that the values being compared should be portrayed side by side. Try different ways of showing the data to see which figure makes the point most clearly. However, do this in pencil first, before spending a few hours with a computer. Three-dimensional graphs are usually not helpful. For example, consider a graph showing the probability of intensive care unit admission by age and sex. Given that there are three dimensions to the data (age, sex, and the probability of admission), the first temptation may be to create a fancy three-dimensional graph such as Figure 7-13.

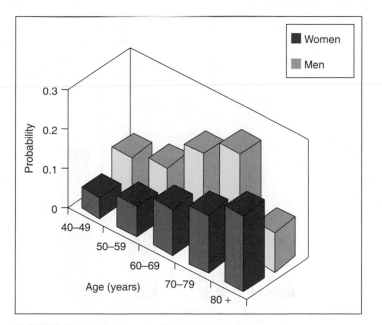

FIGURE 7-13. Likelihood of admission to an intensive care unit (as a proportion of all hospital admissions) by age and sex

But a plain two-dimensional bar graph can demonstrate the same results with less clutter, as Figure 7-14 shows.

A little more tinkering eliminates extraneous lines and rearranges the bars so that the taller one in each pair stands to the right in most cases, in keeping with the overall trend in the figure (Fig. 7-15).

Three-dimensional graphs are sometimes appropriate if you have more than two categories to display for more than one variable. For example, in plotting

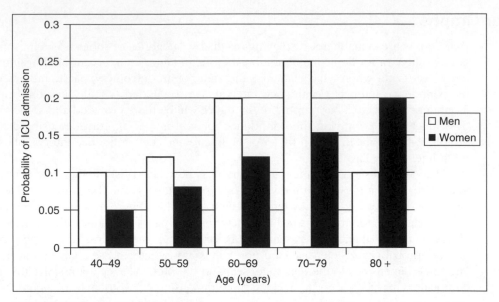

FIGURE 7-14. Likelihood of admission to an intensive care unit (as a proportion of all hospital admissions) by age and sex

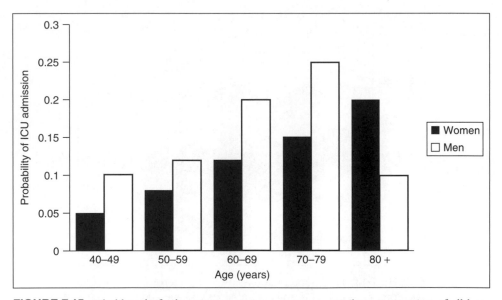

FIGURE 7-15. Likelihood of admission to an intensive care unit (as a proportion of all hospital admissions) by age and sex

the risk of hepatoma in 16 categories of age and alcohol consumption, a three-dimensional graph can indicate that the risk increases continuously with age and alcohol consumption (Fig. 7-16). A two-dimensional graph can be almost as, and often even more, effective (Fig. 7-17).

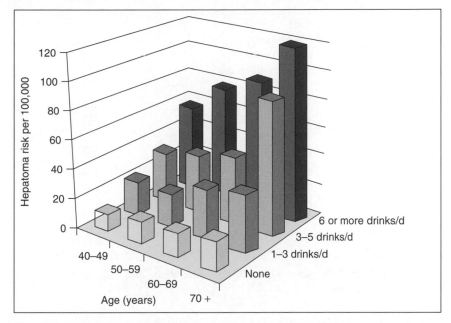

FIGURE 7-16. Annual risk of hepatoma by age and daily alcohol consumption

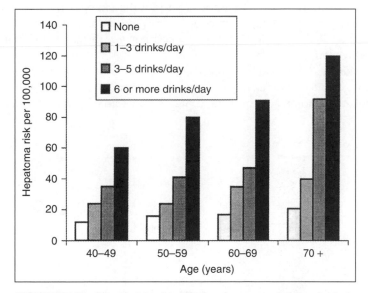

FIGURE 7-17. Annual risk of hepatoma by age and daily alcohol consumption

When the pattern is clear, there is no need to use crosshatched or lined bars to distinguish categories; they just make the figure look busy (Fig. 7-18). If the pattern is not clear, use white, black, hatched gray, and darkly speckled gray (as in Fig. 7-22). Keep the different types of bars to no more than four or five.

Stacked bar graphs, such as the numbers of cases of a disease in different hospitals, can be hard to understand if there are more than a few categories being stacked. Often, a table works better for this kind of data. There are a few exceptions,

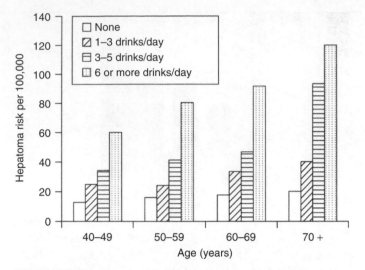

FIGURE 7-18. Annual risk of hepatoma by age and daily alcohol consumption

such as if the bars represent data that sum to the same quantity (e.g., 100%). Suppose, for example, that you are graphing choice of primary care residency programs among fourth-year medical students at three different times. At each time, the various causes sum to 100%. Bar graphs that plot the changes by time within each type of residency or the changes in choices by time do not convey this message very clearly (Fig. 7-19 and Fig. 7-20). A stacked bar graph makes the point much more effectively (Fig. 7-21).

Stacked bar graphs also work if there is a natural order to categorical data that can be exploited. For example, if you are comparing where patients die (in the hospital or at home) in the United States and Canada, there is a natural order to

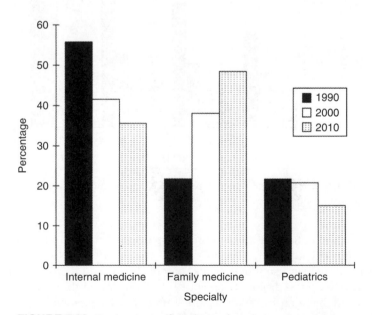

FIGURE 7-19. Proportions of students choosing various primary care specialties in 1990, 2000, and 2010

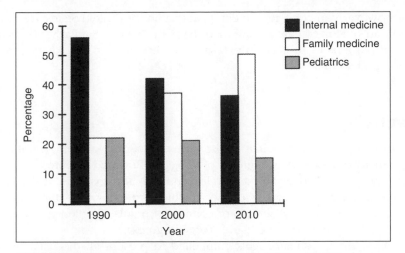

FIGURE 7-20. Proportions of students in 1990, 2000, and 2010 choosing various primary care specialties

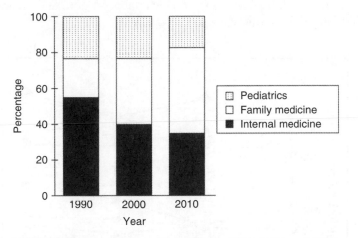

FIGURE 7-21. Proportions of students in 1990, 2000, and 2010 choosing various primary care specialties

the possibilities (died in an intensive care unit, died in a hospital, died in a nursing home, or died at home). A simple stacked bar graph such as Figure 7-22 clarifies

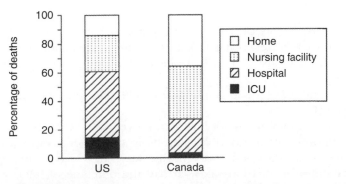

FIGURE 7-22. Site of death among persons 65 years of age and older in the United States and in Canada, 2008

that however you consider the data, patients in the United States are more likely to die in an organized care setting than those in Canada. Similarly, you could portray the proportions of subjects in two groups who have no risk factors, only one risk factor, and so on.

Line Graphs

Because they connect points, line graphs are terrific at demonstrating what has happened to a subject or a group of subjects. Beware of overcrowding the figure with open and filled diamonds, circles, squares, and triangles. If the reader has to constantly refer back to a key to discern which group is which, the main point of the figure may be lost. Four groups of connected points are plenty; if you have more, consider using two or more figures (or subfigures).

Often, an investigator feels compelled to present all the data that have been collected (e.g., diastolic blood pressure in 10 subjects, by time). The resultant figure looks like a "spaghetti" graph, with strands going in many directions (Fig. 7-23). Unless the purpose of the figure is to convey confusion or to tease readers into looking for a hidden message, these should be avoided.

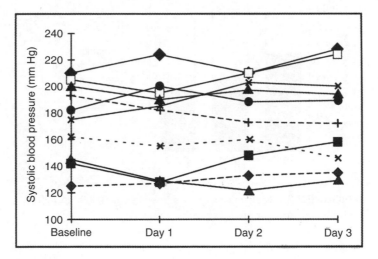

FIGURE 7-23. Blood pressure in 10 subjects treated with ineffectivipine

Never use points or dots to portray nondata points, such as confidence intervals or projected rates. Points (squares, triangles, etc.) should always indicate data-derived observations; Figure 7-24 illustrates a figure that should *not* appear in a manuscript.

If you are using a line graph for a model, then present the modeled lines with error bars (Fig. 7-25).

Another common type of line graph involves survival curves that demonstrate what proportion of a group of subjects is still alive at various times (Fig. 7-26). Sometimes these curves show event-free survival, which is the proportion of study subjects still alive that have not yet had the outcome of interest, say, a hip fracture (these are sometimes known as *Kaplan–Meier curves*). Always include the

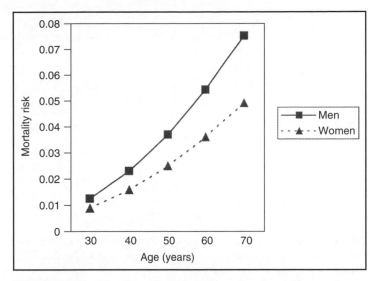

FIGURE 7-24. Mortality risk modeled as a function of age and sex

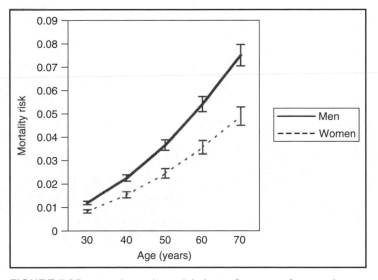

FIGURE 7-25. Mortality risk modeled as a function of age and sex. Error bars indicate 95% confidence intervals for modeled risk

denominators at risk at the various time points. Be sure that the periods make sense (e.g., months or years); if you let a statistics program decide the scale for the *x* axis, you can get a strange choice, such as 0 to 165 days of follow-up, in 5 units of 33 days each.

A bar and whisker plot is a useful type of figure for describing the distribution of data. Such figures can be used to show the range, mean, median, and 25th and 75th percentiles for continuous variables; other attributes (mode, 95% confidence interval for the mean and 10th and 90th percentiles) can also be added (Fig. 7-27).

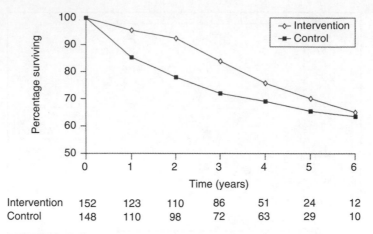

Intervention	152	123	110	86	51	24	12
Control	148	110	98	72	63	29	10

FIGURE 7-26. Cancer recurrence-free survival comparing the intervention and control groups during a 6-year follow-up. The denominators for each group are indicated

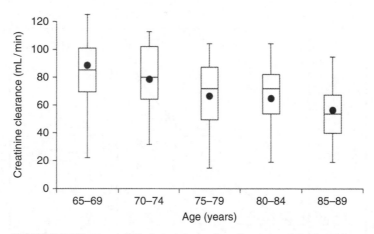

FIGURE 7-27. Mean (filled circle), median (horizontal line), 25th and 75th percentiles (box), and range (whiskers) of creatinine clearance by age of the subjects

---

FIGURE LEGENDS AND TEXT

Figures can accommodate a surprising amount of text. Along with the legend for the figure itself (e.g., Figure. Rate of melanoma by hours of exposure to sunlight among Australian surfers), there are the labels for the abscissa (the *x* axis: average daily sunlight exposure in hours), the ordinate (the *y* axis: melanoma rates/100,000 person years), and the bars or lines (white is men and black is women). Sometimes, *P* values and the *N*s of events or subjects are included. Overcrowding is undesirable, but inadequate documentation is worse. Remember that if your article is well received, the figure may be reproduced as a slide, or for a handout, by many of your readers. Take the time to get it right.

The legend describes what is in the figure. (Many spreadsheet programs use the term *legend* to refer to the key for the figure and use the term *title* for the figure legend.) The legend should not give away the results but should be an objective description of the contents of the figure:

Tells the Answer:

Figure 1 Survival was greater in subjects treated with savopril than in controls

More Objective:

Figure 1 Two-year survival among patients with analgesic nephropathy treated with savopril or placebo

Include enough information so that the reader can understand the figure easily:

The dotted line represents the treatment group; the solid line represents the control.

Even better, label the lines directly or include a key within the figure that indicates what each line or shading represents.

Just as with tables, avoid ambiguous abbreviations, such as "Group 1." Readers should be able to understand the point of the figure at a glance. They will not be able to do so if they have to refer to a key or to the legend to decipher your code.

Usually, a figure legend is too short to include all the important points that a figure conveys. Use the text to complement it. Once again, avoid sentences such as "Figure 1 shows…." Instead, mention the finding, followed by a parenthetical pointer to the figure: "The risk of hepatoma increased with age and alcohol use, such that those older than age 70 years who drank heavily were at more than 10 times the risk of men less than age 40 years who did not drink (Fig. 1)."

SUBMITTING FIGURES WITH A MANUSCRIPT

Figures usually look better in published articles than they do in manuscript form. This problem is exacerbated because some journals specify that the figure legends be included on a separate sheet of paper. This is for the convenience of the typesetters or their computer-age replacements who will eventually be preparing the manuscript for publication, if it is accepted. Having a stack of your figures, with the legends on a separate page, however, is inconvenient for the reviewers and editors, who cannot tell which figure is which, or the legend that goes with a particular figure. The review process involves shuffling back and forth between the text, the figure legends, and the figures themselves. Therefore, place each legend below the appropriate figure as it will eventually appear in the journal, one figure and legend per page (see Chapter 9 on electronic publishing for further advice on how to package your final manuscript).

For figures that you submit as photographs, type the legend on a label and attach it to the back of the photograph, with an up arrow indicating the correct direction. That way, the reviewer will be able to flip the glossy over to see what it is supposed to be about. But a digital version, with the legend underneath, will usually be much better.

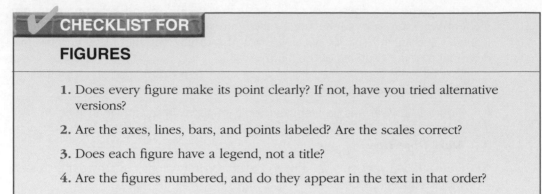

CHECKLIST FOR

FIGURES

1. Does every figure make its point clearly? If not, have you tried alternative versions?

2. Are the axes, lines, bars, and points labeled? Are the scales correct?

3. Does each figure have a legend, not a title?

4. Are the figures numbered, and do they appear in the text in that order?

5. Does the text complement the information in the figures?

8 Discussion

Writing the discussion should be the least stressful part of creating your manuscript. You are in the home stretch. The data have been collected and analyzed, and the Methods and Results sections have probably been written. All that remains is to provide some commentary on your study, which should be a piece of cake. After all, who knows more about what your results mean than you do?

However, why is writing the Discussion section a stumbling block for many investigators? Perhaps because doing so evokes feelings reminiscent of the terror they felt writing an essay for a college-level English class. Panic sets in, and the all-too-common result becomes a dull Discussion section, in which the author reiterates the findings, lists a bunch of previous studies in the area, mentions a few limitations of the current study, repeats the results, and tacks on an insipid conclusion:

> We found X in our study of 284 subjects. Previously, Elhanan et al. studied 123 patients, and found Y. Brown, in a report based on 45 patients, showed Z. Our study had a few limitations, including A, B, and C. In conclusion, we observed X. Our findings may have clinical importance. Further research is needed.

Can you imagine writing, or have you ever actually written, either of the previous two sentences? If so, read on, because help is on the way.

If you are having difficulty writing the discussion, start by imagining that someone else did your study, and you have been asked to comment about it. That will encourage you to look at your results with fresh eyes. Ask yourself the following questions: What did the study show? What might that mean? How else could the results be interpreted? Have other studies had similar results, or is there disagreement in the field? What are this study's strengths and weaknesses? What are the clinical or scientific implications of the results? What, exactly, should happen next in this field of research?

Scrutinize a few good articles in your research area to see what sorts of points are covered in the discussions. Especially in the more prestigious journals, the discussion section may have been rewritten three or four times to satisfy the reviewers and editors and then edited carefully by a professional. Looking at these will help you acquire a sense of the main issues in the field.

Make a brief outline (or at least a list) of the four to six points that you want to cover in the discussion (beyond just repeating the results, which does not count). There may be other topics that you want to add in subsequent revisions, but start with what matters most and build the Discussion section around those points. Here is an example of such a list:

> Health care costs were about 25% greater in diabetic patients who developed new proteinuria than in those with persistently normal urinalyses.

> We had excellent follow-up, which may have explained why we found a difference when no one else has.
>
> Our findings suggest that physicians should monitor urinary protein excretion in diabetic patients at least annually.
>
> There was no practical difference between using a urinary dipstick and more exact measurement techniques because the improvement in precision was counterbalanced by a decreased frequency of measurement.
>
> Although based on a small sample, we observed similar results among patients who did not speak English.

Once you have figured out what you want to say, the challenge becomes explaining and then linking your thoughts so that readers are not bombarded with a series of random impressions. *This is hard work and comes naturally to few scientists.* Perhaps that explains why we chose medicine instead of journalism. Relax. Your college English professor will not be grading your work. Actually, no one will be, if that is any consolation! If you still cannot get started, look under the heading, "Putting It All Together," near the end of this chapter, for some hints about ways to organize and link your paragraphs.

Journal editors do not award a prize for the longest discussion of the year, so keep the discussion terse. A few good paragraphs will suffice. Extraneous material will just be distracting.

STRUCTURE

The discussion should cover a few basic topics, including what you found, what you think your results mean, how your results compare with those of prior studies, and the limitations of your study. A concluding paragraph should highlight the key findings, and your recommendations about what should happen next.

As you become more comfortable writing Discussion sections, you can vary this general formula. For example, suppose your study was a clinical trial showing that treatment of low back pain with a heating pad for 30 minutes a day was more effective than bed rest. The results and their interpretation are straightforward, so there may be no need to repeat them. Instead, you can begin by mentioning the context—the many previous studies of treatments for back pain—in which your study took place.

If your study answers a particularly controversial question, you may want to start the discussion by outlining the history of the controversy. If you are reversing previous dogma, you may want to summarize the evidence behind it. But in a pinch, when faced with an empty page or computer screen and no clue about how to begin, follow the tried-and-true formula in this chapter.

WHAT YOU FOUND

Begin with the key finding of your study. Synthesize and summarize—do not simply reiterate the exact results. Use words rather than numbers. If you must use numbers, keep them simple. Here are some examples of opening sentences:

> A nonpharmacologic intervention to reduce blood pressure resulted in improved quality of life among patients who had previously been treated with β-blockers.

When compared with age-matched controls, children with frequent episodes of bronchitis were about twice as likely to develop symptomatic hearing loss.

Patients with advanced colon cancer who were treated with endothelial vascular relaxation factor had a 4-month longer median survival than those treated with placebo.

If appropriate, provide a common metric for the reader:

The increase in stroke risk associated with a 10% decline in serum albumin is similar to that associated with a 15 mm Hg increase in systolic blood pressure.

Next, mention other findings that were important, using a similar approach. However, do not present any results for the first time in the discussion. All results should debut in the Results section with appropriate methods in the Methods section.

WHAT YOU THINK THE RESULTS MEAN AND HOW STRONGLY YOU BELIEVE THEM

In the part of the discussion where you interpret your results and indicate how convincing you find them, you are telling readers why your results matter. Your interpretation of the results should depend on how successfully you can convince yourself that alternative interpretations are less valid. That, in turn, depends on the careful consideration of those alternatives. Sharing this thought process with the readers should constitute a large part of the discussion. Consider all the implications of your results, whether clinical, biologic, methodologic, economic, or ethical.

These results indicate that clinicians should consider the use of endovaginal ultrasound in all patients with a family history of endometrial cancer.

Our findings may have important biologic implications, in that they point out the possibility that infectious particles may not contain DNA or RNA.

This study emphasizes the feasibility of enrolling subjects who are unwilling to volunteer for standard clinical trials.

Indicate the strength of your convictions. Are you certain, nearly certain, 50/50, or just playing a hunch?

These findings demonstrate that effective therapy for advanced melanoma is a reality.

Our results suggest that effective therapy for advanced melanoma is possible.

A reasonable interpretation of these results is that effective therapies for advanced melanoma can be developed.

Based on our results, it is at least theoretically possible that an effective therapy for advanced melanoma will be developed.

Although it is worthwhile to mention a study's strengths and unique features, do not brag, especially by claiming that yours is the first study to have made a particular accomplishment:

This is the first study to have prospectively assessed changes in mood in a cohort of adolescent boys from Nebraska. Previous studies have used a retrospective design among children from the other 49 states.

Priority claims, such as "This is the first (or largest, or best) study" have a way of annoying reviewers, especially since such claims are often wrong. You will be in a better position if the reviewers (and readers) make that judgment for themselves.

Some findings do not require much explanation. If you found that 10% of your subjects wore contact lenses, there is not much to say about that finding. Similarly, a well-done randomized trial that shows that one treatment works better and costs less than another may not need a lot of fancy explanations.

Extrapolate from your data. Suppose you showed that 187 of the 925 subjects in your study complained of back pain and that your sample was reasonably representative of a larger population. Then you might write something like:

> About one in five men and women of ages 15 to 64 years reported back pain in the past 12 months. If these results are applicable to the almost 200 million US adults in this age group, they would indicate that about 40 million of these Americans suffer from back pain each year.

Avoid appearing silly by being unrealistically precise:

> We found that 20.2% of men and women of ages 15 to 64 years reported back pain. Applying these results to the 198,238,509 US adults between the ages of 15 and 64 years, we estimate that 40,076,326 Americans in this age group suffer from back pain each year.

Associations in Analytic Studies

Analytic results—those that involve the association between two or more variables—from nonrandomized studies usually benefit from an explanation. (If you are not sure whether you have done an analytic study, see Chapter 5.) If you have done an analytic study and have found an association between a predictor variable and an outcome variable, remember that there are five potential explanations for that association: *chance, bias, effect–cause, effect–effect,* and *cause–effect.* Each of these possibilities usually deserves discussion. Suppose, for example, that you have done a study looking at whether inflammation, as measured by the erythrocyte sedimentation rate (ESR), is associated with the risk of stroke. Your results show that an elevated ESR is associated with an increased risk of stroke (relative risk = 2.0, with a 95% confidence interval from 1.2 to 3.2; $P = 0.01$). It is worth exploring each of the five possible explanations for the ESR–stroke association in more detail.

Chance defines something that happens without a discernible, predictable cause (e.g., someone wins the lottery every month, and it is impossible to venture which ticket holder is likelier to win than any other). We evaluate the likelihood that chance is the explanation for a finding by doing statistical tests. (For more on confidence intervals and P values, see Chapter 5.) In the example about ESR and stroke, the P value is small, and the confidence interval excludes no effect. Thus, chance is not a particularly likely explanation for the results, especially because the hypothesis was stated in advance.

When evaluating the possibility of chance, investigators have a tendency to be foolish. They often ignore an association with a P value of 0.06 and overemphasize an association with a P value of 0.04. Most statisticians (but all too few journal editors and reviewers) recognize that there is nothing magical about P values <0.05.

Bias results from inadvertent mistakes in the design or execution of the study. (If the mistakes are intentional, they are called *fraud,* which is, unfortunately, another potential explanation for an association.) Perhaps the sample in the study of ESR and stroke was chosen from a group of patients with an unusually high prevalence of vasculitis. Maybe the physicians caring for patients with high ESRs were more likely to order brain-imaging studies and consequently more subclinical strokes were diagnosed.

Some study designs are susceptible to subtle forms of bias. A study of a chronic problem that waxes and wanes and that uses patients as their controls can be susceptible to bias owing to *regression to the mean*. That is, if patients with rheumatoid arthritis are enrolled in a study when they are in the midst of an arthritis flare, almost any therapy will appear to be effective unless it is compared with a placebo. *Recall bias* occurs when subjects with a condition are more likely to remember certain aspects of their history than healthy controls. This often affects studies that rely on subjects' self-reports. More generally, any study in which variables are not ascertained blindly and objectively can be biased.

For the first two explanations of association—bias and chance—the association that you found in your study is not actually real. It was a by-product of your research design or analysis or a result of bad luck. The other three explanations—effect–cause, effect–effect, and cause–effect—involve associations that are real. But only the last of these (cause–effect) implies that the predictor causes the outcome.

Effect–cause means that the outcome causes the predictor; for example, a stroke causes the ESR to rise. More subtly, perhaps the inflammation associated with subclinical strokes causes an increase in the ESR.

Effect–effect occurs when another process causes both the predictor and the outcome. This situation sometimes goes by the epidemiologic name of *confounding*. In the example, perhaps age causes the ESR to rise, and age causes strokes. Age is said to confound the association between ESR and stroke. While there are many multivariate statistical techniques for adjusting for confounders, one can only adjust for those that have been considered and measured. If a confounder was not measured, or was measured poorly, one cannot adjust for it.

Cause–effect, in which the predictor causes the outcome, is the easiest association to explain. It is also the explanation an investigator usually wants to establish. In the example, a high ESR actually causes stroke. This example, however, points out a problem with cause–effect. Sometimes it just does not make good sense. After all, an abnormal laboratory test cannot "cause" a stroke. Many well-accepted cause–effect associations, such as that between male sex and coronary heart disease, or between advanced age and many diseases, presumably result from some undetermined factor or factors.

There are other criteria that are sometimes applied when one is assessing whether an association is causal. Some, such as whether the cause preceded the effect, are reasonably obvious. Others, such as whether the association makes biologic sense, are not very useful. People are good at concocting plausible explanations for just about anything, and sometimes an apparently ridiculous explanation (prions or *Helicobacter pylori*, for example) turns out to be correct. Another criterion—that of a dose–response relation between the cause and the effect—does not distinguish among the other explanations. After all, "the more effect, the more cause."

A key reason why blinded, randomized, controlled trials have become the standard for evaluating the effects of a treatment is that they deal effectively with several of the alternative explanations if you find an association. In these studies, the cause is the intervention—as compared with the control—and the effect is the main outcome of the trial. Randomly assigning patients to a treatment group and to a control group deals with several problems. Having a control group makes it unlikely that regression to the mean (patients getting better on their own) can explain the results. Assuming that both groups are treated identically, bias is unlikely. If the groups are similar at the beginning of the trial, based on attributes that can be measured, it is unlikely that some unmeasured confounder will differ between the groups. Therefore, effect–effect is unlikely. The structure of the trial makes effect–cause impossible because the outcome cannot determine to which group a participant had previously been randomly assigned. Therefore, at the end of the study, the only possible explanations are chance, whose likelihood can be estimated statistically, and cause–effect.

Actually, there is one important alternative that needs to be considered—co-interventions that happen to the intervention group (or the controls) that were not part of the planned intervention. Consider a successful randomized trial of the effect of diet on heart disease. The investigators will not be able to conclude that the dietary intervention was successful if it turned out that those in the diet group were more likely to start exercising because there were sign-up lists for exercise training at the nutritionists' offices.

What If You Did an Analytic Study and Did Not Find an Association?

There are several potential explanations for failing to find an effect in your study. A few of these reasons parallel those for finding an association.

Lack of power and imprecision in measurements are almost always potential explanations for failing to find an association. *Power* is a statistical term for the likelihood of finding an effect of a given size or larger in your study, if the effect is actually present in the real world. You can lack power because you did not have enough subjects with outcomes or if you did not have enough subjects with the predictor variable of interest. That can happen with a rare disease or with an unusual exposure, even if the total number of subjects in the study was large. For example, a study of 5,000 middle-aged subjects would probably lack power to detect the risk factors for Wegener granulomatosis (because it is a very rare disease); it would also lack sufficient power to detect whether subjects who wore hearing aids were at greater risk of motor vehicle accidents.

Besides inadequate sample size, imprecision in measurement can also cause a lack of power. If the predictor or outcome variables were measured poorly, that causes what is called *nondifferential misclassification*. (The word *nondifferential* means that the misclassification happens at random.) A study that ascertained the presence of diabetes by self-report would misclassify many elderly subjects. Non-differential misclassification reduces power to detect associations in the same way that a smeared lens reduces the sharpness of a photograph. The information may be there; it is just harder to make it out. Similarly, *invalid* measurements—in which what you actually measured does not adequately represent what you think you measured—also make it harder to find an effect. For example, a study of jaundice in newborns that relies on physical examination rather than on the serum bilirubin concentration may yield erroneous results.

Finally, problems with power can occur if there are a lot of *missing data,* especially if multivariable analysis techniques are used. Unless special techniques are used to "impute" (a fancy word for "make an educated guess about") the missing values, then subjects who are missing data about *any* of the variables in the model will be excluded. Sometimes, the actual number of subjects in a multivariable model is only half, or less, of the total number in your sample.

It is also possible to have *reverse confounding*, in which you do not find an effect in your sample because you did not adjust for important variables. Had you done so, the effect would have been apparent. For example, your study might find that estrogen use in women is not associated with heart disease. Although there was no net effect of estrogen, a more complete analysis might have found that estrogen use was associated with a decreased risk in women without heart disease but an increased risk in women who have heart disease.

Of course, you will probably not find an effect in your study if it is correct, and there is actually no effect in the real world. But proving the absence of an effect is usually a process of exclusion. You must convince the reviewers that your measurements were valid and that the 95% confidence intervals for the key results were sufficiently narrow to excuse a substantial effect. Suppose you studied the effect of living near electric power lines on the incidence of childhood leukemia and found no effect. You found that children who lived within 50 meters of power lines had an odds ratio of 1.1 for leukemia with a 95% confidence interval from 0.8 to 1.5. Therefore, the results of your study are inconsistent with exposure to electric power lines being responsible for a 2-fold increase in risk. Although the results could not exclude a relatively minor increase (say, a 1.4-fold to 1.5-fold greater risk), that sort of increased risk is probably not very meaningful, especially for a rare disease such as leukemia. However, if a study had an odds ratio of 1.1 with a 95% confidence interval from 0.2 to 5.5, the study will not be able to exclude even a 5-fold increased risk.

Finally, negative results can be the consequence of poor design, execution, or analysis. This perhaps explains why it can be difficult to get a study with negative results published, particularly if the reviewers or editors have any concerns about the quality of the study. If you are at the manuscript preparation stage, there is not much you can do about how a study was designed and executed, but you can at least make sure that you have done the best possible job analyzing and presenting the negative findings.

SECONDARY RESULTS

When discussing secondary results, treat them as you did your primary results—synthesize and summarize rather than simply repeat what you found:

> We also found that the improvement in quality of life was greatest in those who reported good or excellent relationships with their physicians.

> Our study also showed that the *neu* oncogene was not associated with prognosis in patients with digestive tract cancers.

Do not avoid your difficult secondary results, such as those that were surprising, did not make sense, or were found in one part of the sample but not in another. If you can explain why a set of results appears internally contradictory, it is almost always worth taking the time to do so. If you cannot, then say so:

> We were surprised to find that tea drinking was associated with cancer of the pancreatic islets.

> It is possible that this is a true association, but this may also be a chance result.

> Tea contains several substances that have been associated with gastric tumors in rodents.

> We cannot explain why tea drinking should cause malignant islet cell tumors.

Never speculate if you have the data:

> One possible explanation for our results is that the tea drinkers in our study were more likely to have a family history of endocrine tumors than those who did not drink tea.

Well, did they? This is a simple question to answer.

Not every result warrants comment. Refrain from discussing results that are self-explanatory or common knowledge:

> In our study of patients with diabetes and hypercholesterolemia, there were more deaths from heart disease than from lightning strikes.

> Chronic otitis media was associated with an increased risk of hearing loss.

Sometimes, if you have several important results to discuss, you may want to group them—first, all the findings—then, all the interpretations. At other times, it makes more sense to discuss each result and its interpretation separately and finishing with one finding before moving on to the next one.

HOW DO YOUR RESULTS COMPARE WITH PRIOR KNOWLEDGE?

Synthesize the results of prior studies. How does your study expand on those studies? Do not review the entire literature. Pick the most important prior studies and reference some of the other good ones:

> Some (1–3), but not all (4–7), previous studies have found that... Fleming, for example, ...(5)

Occasionally, it may be more efficient to use a table to summarize the main features of several previous studies.

If the results of your study disagree with what other investigators have found, attempt to explain why. Do your results actually differ, or do they overlap with other findings in a statistical sense? Are there important differences in the design of the studies, the characteristics of subjects, or the way measurements were made?

> Although our results may seem to differ with those of Baldwin et al., we used a different method of ascertaining compliance with therapy than they did.

> Our findings are consistent with those of Kay and Rugen, given the wide confidence intervals in both studies.

Do not harp on limitations of other research, as the authors may be assigned to review your study. Be gently critical by being factual:

> In their study, Best et al. concluded that larger doses of nonsteroidal agents resulted in better analgesia, but they did not evaluate the statistical significance of their results.

> Sander and colleagues did not obtain EKGs or troponin levels; they ascertained myocardial infarction by self-report.

> Low reported preliminary results, in abstract form, in 11 patients.

Avoid the temptation to write a paragraph about each of the dozen or so previous studies in your subject area. If there are a few seminal studies, describe them in more detail. If there is no relevant literature, do not feel obliged to dredge something up just for the appearance of completeness.

If you wrote your article primarily for a scientific audience, spend some time discussing the clinical implications of the results. If you are writing for a clinical audience, do not ignore the scientific significance of your work. The medical literature may be written mainly by academic physicians, but it is read by clinicians in practice and people with PhDs working in laboratories. Your work will have a greater impact if you can make all of these groups appreciate it.

LIMITATIONS OF THE STUDY

Every study has its problems. You must identify those that may affect the validity or meaning of your study. Discussing the limitations of your study serves several purposes. First, it forces you to critique your work. By doing so, you may improve your understanding of the results. Second, a clear assessment of the weaknesses of your study indicates to a reviewer that you are an objective scientist who understands research. Finally, a discussion of the limitations of a study helps the reader to understand the important methodologic points in the field, such as potential biases, and the importance of adequate power.

Sometimes, you cannot think of any limitations. For example, you may have done a randomized, double-blinded, placebo-controlled study of 150,000 patients of all ages from 10 countries on four continents with total mortality as the endpoint and no loss to follow-up during the 15-year study. Congratulations. In that case, you may simply write, "Our study had no limitations" and skip the rest of this section. But every other study (hint: including yours) has its limitations. If you cannot think of any, ask, "If I could do the study over, what changes will I make?" For example, was the design sufficiently rigorous? Were the subjects appropriate? Were the measurements precise and valid? Was the follow-up complete? Were the analyses properly done? Were all potential outcomes and confounders measured? What was not done that might have been useful?

Do not just list the limitations—explain them. In this regard, familiarity with the field may get in your way. Do not assume that everyone reading your article will know why it matters that you selected your sample from volunteers; that some of the measurements were made with an out-of-date technology; or that you did not use a logistic regression model to analyze the data. Say why you think each particular limitation matters:

> We studied volunteer nurses and physical therapists, who had very high rates of compliance with the treatment. Therefore, we likely overestimated the benefits of the treatment in actual practice.

> We measured plasma porcelain titers using the Kahn–Crete method, which is less reliable than the technology recently developed by Khotani.

> We were unable to fit a logistic regression model to our data, probably because of the small number of outcomes.

Sometimes, limitations are imposed by external conditions, such as lack of funds:

> One limitation of our study is that serum samples were obtained only once. We did not have sufficient resources to make more frequent measurements, which may have provided more meaningful information.

Consider all the potential limitations of your study, from design to interpretation. Many investigators ignore the issue of limitations in their interpretation of the results. Instead, they concentrate on discussing how their sample might have been bigger or more representative or how they could have used a more precise method of making one of the measurements. But being critical of how you have interpreted your results is just as essential.

> Our results could also be interpreted as showing that therapy with calcium is ineffective in preventing osteoporosis. Although bone density was increased, fracture rates were no different than in the control group.

> Although the differences we observed were statistically significant, they were generally small and may not be clinically meaningful.

> We found that patients with nephrotic syndrome had a greater incidence of pulmonary embolism than the normal controls. However, when the rates of pulmonary embolism observed in this study were compared with those in the literature for other patients with hypercoagulable states, pulmonary embolism was actually less common than might have been expected.

It is often helpful to make a list of your major findings and what you think they mean. Then consider other ways someone might interpret them. Why is your interpretation better?

Do not overdo the limitations. Worse than belittling someone else's study is harping on your own study's shortcomings. Mention how you dealt with potential limitations and balance them with the study's strengths. If you believe that a particular limitation is not important, do not be afraid to say so.

> Although this was a prospective study, it has several limitations. We were unable to measure all potential confounders, including....

> The study took place in a single medical center; although patients were drawn from a variety of ethnic groups and socioeconomic backgrounds, we cannot determine....

> Follow-up data were not available for six subjects; however, even if we assumed that all of them died it would not affect our overall conclusions.

CONCLUSIONS AND IMPLICATIONS

Imagine you are looking the reader in the eye. What is your take-home message? How should your results change the reader's beliefs or actions?

> These results emphasize the value of periodic foot examinations in nondiabetic patients with peripheral neuropathy. Patients should have a thorough examination each year. Those with evidence of peripheral vascular disease need to be examined more frequently, at least every 6 months.

> Loss of the short arm of chromosome 13 is associated with a poor prognosis in patients with melanoma. Examination of the chromosomal pattern should

be a routine part of prognostic staging of the disease. Further investigations to determine the biologic mechanism through which loss of the alleles on this chromosome affects prognosis may suggest novel methods of treatment or prevention.

You can compare your results with other studies or combine your results to generate new implications:

Previous studies have found that foot examinations are beneficial in patients with diabetes. Along with our results in patients with nondiabetic neuropathy, this suggests that neuropathy, per se, rather than just diabetes, is associated with the development of foot ulcers.

Clark's grade has long been used in staging melanoma. The chromosomal pattern, specifically deletion of the short arm of chromosome 13, provides additional prognostic information.

Do not be a wimp. You are now an expert. Take a position:

Despite the limitations of our study, and the weight of scientific evidence since Columbus, we believe our results are most consistent with the hypothesis that the Earth is flat. Our results also provide the first inklings of evidence in favor of intelligent design.

(Okay, maybe it is not worth taking a position as extreme as this last one!)

Do not just end by recommending additional research or by pleading ignorance. Never use any of these sentences:

Additional research is needed.

Our findings may have clinical significance.

Further studies to confirm these findings would be helpful.

The meaning of these results is uncertain.

If you feel compelled in this direction, at least make some specific suggestions:

Future research should follow patients for a longer period, at least 5 years, and validate outcomes radiographically.

Studies of patients earlier in the course of the disease, before the onset of respiratory symptoms, would be enlightening.

A randomized trial comparing these two therapies, with complete cessation of blood loss as the outcome, is needed.

Finally, do not end by repeating the results one last time:

In conclusion, we conclude that we found what we just said we found.

In summary, in the patients we studied, we found our findings.

PUTTING IT ALL TOGETHER

If you write like most people, your discussion will comprise a series of paragraphs, one or two for each of the main parts of the section. Work on having each of those paragraphs make sense (see Chapter 14 for some hints). After you have written these paragraphs, you will be ready to string them together into a coherent discussion section. If you try to write the entire Discussion at once, you may find yourself with too many ideas scattered throughout several pages of text. Editing the mess will be impossible.

After your paragraphs are assembled, think of them as independent units, like pieces of furniture in a room that you are designing. Do not be afraid to move them around to find the right order. Experiment a bit. Should the armchair (limitations) go closer to the fireplace (scientific implications)? Is the couch too big (the paragraph too long)? Maybe the room would be better with two comfortable chairs (short paragraphs) rather than a sofa. Perhaps the end table (a paragraph on prior studies) needs a lamp (a topic sentence). The process of making a whole from the parts requires flexibility.

Then, connect the paragraphs with sentences that segue between ideas:

These results are consistent with....

Our results suggest the possibility that....

After a paragraph on advantages or limitations, you may wish to switch gears:

Our study also had several limitations.

We believe that our results are more reliable than those of Robinski.

Our study also had several strengths. We enrolled more than 200 subjects and had 95% complete follow-up.

Despite these limitations, many of which are inevitable in observational research, we believe that our central conclusions remain valid.

After a paragraph on other results that disagree with yours, explain why there is disagreement:

Why might our results differ? One possibility is that....

These previous studies measured weight in tons, whereas we used a Mettler balance to measure weight in milligrams.

For a paragraph that comes out of the blue, acknowledge your surprise:

We made a number of other observations as well.

Although not previously thought to be related to ..., we also looked at ....

After a dense paragraph lacking clinical utility, bring the reader back to reality:

Our results may have practical importance as well.

While not currently available ....

After a few paragraphs summarizing key studies, tie them together:

What do these studies have in common?

How do these results compare with ours?

When you have completed writing your discussion, review the checklist to see how you have done.

CHECKLIST FOR
DISCUSSION

Title

1. Did you discuss the key findings and explain why they matter?

2. Have you indicated the strength of your convictions?

3. Did you mention alternative interpretations of your results?

4. Have you included the limitations and strengths of the study?

5. Did you make recommendations about what, specifically, should happen next?

6. Did you present any new data from your study? If so, move them to the Results section.

7. Does each paragraph flow from the previous one?

8. Are there trivial points that can be eliminated?

9

References and Electronic Publishing

REFERENCES

Few authors think of their references as a separate part of a manuscript. But they do serve important functions. They demonstrate your familiarity with existing knowledge in the field and direct readers to other literature of interest. Moreover, they provide other investigators with the sources for your methods and furnish editors with a list of potential reviewers, a sense of what other journals have been publishing in the area, and the topicality of the subject matter. If the topic of your manuscript is controversial, your references may disclose whether your conclusions have a particular slant.

A few basic rules apply to using references. First, statements of facts—except those from your present study—must be referenced. However, some facts (e.g., that coronary artery disease is an important health problem) are so obvious that referencing them is silly. So if you are searching for a reference for something that is common knowledge, stop and consider deleting the "fact" from your manuscript and substituting something more interesting.

Second, do not cite a reference that you have not read. Preferably, you should also have a copy of it while you are writing the manuscript. This will prevent the problem of citing the wrong reference for a particular point. For example, you may have read an article that makes a statement ("Black is white.") and provides a reference for that statement. *Never* repeat that statement and reference without verifying its accuracy against the original article. Similarly, do not cite an abstract if the full-length manuscript has been published; indeed, some journals will not let you cite abstracts at all.

Third, have a plan for deciding which references to cite. As a rule, it is more important to cite studies that support the point you are making than those that are "better known" in the field. However, if there are a few (no more than five) truly essential studies, without which the context for your research would not make sense, then cite those as well. Moreover, if you think a reviewer or reader will wonder why you did not cite a study, particularly if the results of the study do not support your point of view, that is a good clue that you need to cite (and discuss!) that study as well.

Fourth, pay attention to the order of references within a sentence and paragraph. Attach references to the appropriate phrase within a sentence ("Some (1–3), but not all (4–7), studies have found that…") so that readers can easily identify which studies support which point. Otherwise, cite references for a particular sentence in chronologic order, beginning with the oldest and ending with the most recent.

Fifth, the Results section should almost never have any reference citations. If you find yourself violating that prohibition, what you are referencing probably belongs either in the Methods or the Discussion section.

Finally, always redo your literature search and references each time you submit, or resubmit, a manuscript. If the reference list is out of date, exceeds the maximum allowed by the journal, or uses a different format than the journal does, reviewers and editors can easily tell that the manuscript has been either rejected several times or gathering dust on your desk.

Background References for the Introduction Section

Choose only a few background references. A recent review of the literature may be preferable to citing 10 or 20 original articles. However, seminal articles—those that were truly groundbreaking—should be cited. If there has not been a review article, provide a succinct summary of the prior literature, including a few references, rather than citing every relevant article.

Some authors mistakenly think that an extensive reference list can substitute for a thorough review of the literature. Merely indicating that you have located pertinent references is not meaningful. You must read them and demonstrate that you understood the implications of each study for your own work.

Methodologic References for the Methods Section

If you have made measurements using an assay, instrument, or questionnaire that has been used previously, cite the original reference. You can then explain the method you used in a sentence or two. If that reference is obscure, however—available only in a specialized library or in a foreign-language journal, for example—provide enough detail in your Methods section so that readers can understand what you did.

If your manuscript is not the first report from your study, cite other references to the study—for instance, one that provides a more detailed description of the sampling or measurement method.

There is a tradition of citing references for statistical tests. For the most part this is not necessary, as most statistical analysis is done with standard software packages. Instead, mention the tests that were used and the software (in case it later turns out that the program had an error or used an invalid statistical method or algorithm). Only if you make a special modification, or are using a technique that is not part of a standard package, should you cite a statistical reference.

Relevant Studies for the Discussion Section

Often, there are hundreds of studies that might be relevant for the Discussion section. Most original articles, however, should have between 20 and 40 references, and you may have already cited 5 or 10 in the Introduction and Methods sections.

Given the plethora of articles you could cite, how should you choose? Keep in mind that most of the Discussion section is exactly that—a discussion of your findings. That part will require no references. You will need to cite prior studies with results that agree or disagree with your own as well as studies that provide a biologic explanation for your results, suggest clinical relevance, or indicate that a similar phenomenon has been observed in other settings or disciplines.

Making a Reference List

There are several bibliography programs for the personal computer that can simplify the process of preparing a reference list. These programs can download and store thousands of references and make them easily available. When writing the manuscript, you simply insert the reference number or a shortened version of the citation (say, author and year) into the text. Subsequently, when you are finished with the manuscript, the program automatically reformats your document, with the citations and reference list included.

You can easily add references to your citation database manually or by downloading the references from a literature search. The latter process reduces but does not eliminate typographic errors. Always check for them. Most electronic references include extraneous material, such as "see comments." Delete these phrases as you download the reference.

Follow the journal's rules about how citations should appear in the text. Some journals prefer that citations be placed in parentheses, others ask for brackets, and others want superscript. Citations should be in numerical order. Use dashes if there are several consecutive references (4–8, not 4,5,6,7,8).

Selective Citations

What about trying to anticipate potential reviewers by citing some of their published work or by citing articles on your subject that have appeared in the journal that you are submitting the manuscript? This strategy ensures that a reviewer is not inadvertently insulted by not being mentioned and may make it more likely that a journal editor will choose that person as a reviewer. It may also help an editor understand why you submitted the manuscript to that particular journal. While reviewers are chosen from a list of experts based on the editors' knowledge of the area, citing particular articles from that journal at least suggests that the authors you are citing would be appropriate reviewers. Be explicit. If there are potential reviewers who have published in that journal, then cite their studies in the references and indicate that you have done so in a cover letter: "Drs. Eric Roberts and David Mangrub have previously published in this area in your journal (References 12 and 16) and are potential reviewers."

Read the Journal's Requirements

Most journals follow a standard reference format, known as the *Vancouver style* because it originated at a meeting of medical journal editors in Vancouver, Canada, in 1978. Guidance on this reference format is provided in the Uniform Requirements for Manuscripts Submitted to Biomedical Journals (see Appendix A). Some journals make minor modifications to the Vancouver style, such as listing journal titles in bold print. You need not do this in your manuscript; the copy editor and publisher will take care of it for you. Other journals have their own reference styles, and you will need to provide your references in the appropriate format. This may not seem important at the time you submit your manuscript, but remember that the more your article looks like it belongs in the targeted journal, the more likely it is to be accepted. Every little bit helps. A bibliographic software program can format your references to the journal's style with a push of a button, which is another reason to use one.

Check your Reference List

Before you submit your manuscript, look over your reference list, especially if you have used a bibliography program. There may be all sorts of odd tidbits. Journal names may have been abbreviated strangely; authors with multiple initials or hyphenated last names may have had their names garbled; and superfluous notes (such as [*see comments*]) may have been inserted. Correct these mistakes before you submit the manuscript. You do not want the reviewers and editors to think that you are a careless scientist. If you did not use a bibliography program, verify each citation against the original article for the spelling of the authors' names; the exact title of the article; and the year, volume, and page numbers. Finally, make sure that the references are cited in the correct order, as they appear in the text.

ELECTRONIC PUBLISHING

Thanks to the Internet, much of the information currently published in journals and books is available instantly and inexpensively. Although the implications of this change for the publishing industry are enormous—for instance, how will the expenses of editing articles and preparing them for publication be covered?—the changes for authors have been less noticeable. The biggest change is that submitting, reviewing, and revising manuscripts have been simplified as journals have moved to electronic submissions. This has somewhat shortened the time needed to process manuscripts and has ensured that manuscripts no longer are in danger of vanishing in the hands of the postal service or overnight delivery services. On the other hand, many scientists now face a weekly barrage of e-mail requests to review articles and have had to memorize all sorts of user names and passwords to access the systems that different journals use. It is definitely a mixed blessing.

Electronic Submission

Nearly all publishing is done electronically, and electronic submission of manuscripts saves time and money for everyone concerned. An electronic copy of a manuscript is either uploaded to a journal's Web site or sent to the journal's e-mail address as an enclosure or attachment. Journals forward the electronic copy of your manuscript, including tables and references, to the journal's publisher for copyediting and preparation for publication. Although many journals can handle electronic versions of cartoons and graphs, figures must sometimes also be submitted in hard copy allowing the editor and publisher to verify the accuracy and completeness of the electronic versions.

Most publishers have software that can convert files from common word-processing programs. If you use an unusual program, consider saving the manuscript as a rich text format file, which is easily opened by most programs; however, formatting of tables and figures may be lost. Whatever program you use, send the documents with a cover note that tells the journal's staff how many tables and figures were sent so that they can confirm their safe arrival.

Manuscript tracing can also be handled electronically, as journals post the current status of submitted manuscripts on their Web sites. This is done by manuscript number so that the whole world will not know what your manuscript is about, or when it was rejected. You simply use a Web browser to locate the journal's Web site by either searching for the journal name or entering the URL (uniform resource locator), which will look something like *http://www.journalname.org*. The http stands for hypertext transfer protocol; the :// is a vestige of UNIX (a computer operating system) code; and www stands for World Wide Web.

If you want to make friends with the office staff at a journal, consider submitting your entire manuscript (abstract, text, references, tables, and figures) as a single PDF document. This will simplify their job. If you do submit your manuscript as several files, be sure that your name (first and last if your name is common) appears in the name of each file that you submit. Even better, also number each file in the correct order in its title (e.g., "1. Baron M. Abstract, text, and references; 2. Baron M. Tables 1–4; 3. Baron M. Figure 1; 4. Baron M. Figure 2."). Once you are given a manuscript number by the editorial office, add that number to the file names.

Like most people, I use Adobe Acrobat for these purposes, and the following instructions refer to that program. There are, of course, other software programs that can accomplish these same tasks. You can find them by searching the Web using the phrase, "Create PDF files." (PDF stands for Portable Document Format.)

If you are going to prepare a PDF file, do the final edits in the word-processing software, and use the PDF maker to compile the final document. Although the PDF maker has a touch-up text tool that can be used to make last minute edits, it is not easy to use. If you do make touch-up changes in the PDF version, make the same changes in the source materials also.

Be sure to delete all the page numbers (and headers and footers) from the original documents. Otherwise, they will show up in the PDF file and will almost certainly be wrong. You can easily add page numbers to the final PDF version.

The key command is "Create PDF" from the File menu, using the "from Multiple Files" option if you are going to combine several files (e.g., the word-processed text of the manuscript, plus the tables, plus the figures, etc.) into a single PDF file. Use the Browse function to find the files you want to include. Then select and add them to the list. You can arrange them in the desired order for the final document by highlighting each file and moving it up (or down). Then push the OK button and wait a few minutes while your PDF document is created. Eventually, you will have to give the final version a name, such as, "Your name. The first few words of the manuscript title." After making your PDF file, you can often compress it further, using the PDF optimizer option in the Advanced menu.

Watch out for the Attach command—it is probably not something you want to do.

Making a PDF file adds a few minutes to the overall process of preparing a manuscript for submission. However, it should be fun, as no writing is involved!

You can also use the security feature to ensure that no one can make changes to (or copy) your document. Be aware, however, that the journal office that receives your document will need to copy it. Finally, do not worry about the "bookmarks" that the PDF maker creates. They are not relevant for manuscript review or publication.

Journal Web Sites

Electronic publishing has another purpose. Documents can be linked, so that clicking on a key word or reference takes the reader to another Web site. As more journals develop Web sites, articles in your reference list can be linked to the one that contains the text of that citation. Articles published in journals recognized by the National Library of Medicine get a unique identifier number that ensures linking even if an author's name is misspelled. Including these identifiers and links, however, currently takes some extra effort. Many Web sites include a search engine, in which an interested visitor enters a term and then is provided with links to each article on that site that contains the term of interest.

As more journals become available on the Web, it will become possible to see the abstracts, and often even the full text, of the references in your bibliography. This is another reason to make sure that the cited reference says what you claimed.

Few investigators will be made responsible for converting a manuscript into a Web-friendly document that can link to other references or sites, in hypertext markup language (HTML). Publishers will handle this task. However, many common word-processing programs can save manuscripts in HTML format, and preparing Web-ready documents is being taught in many elementary schools.

Nonjournal Web Sites

Getting a manuscript accepted for publication usually involves a long process of peer review, whereas anyone with a homepage or who knows someone with a homepage can post information on the Web instantaneously. The Web is not peer reviewed, however. If you are participating in a nonstandard site, a few caveats apply. Suppose, for example, that you have done a study on laryngeal cancer, and someone asks you to post that information on his or her cancer care Web site. Should you agree to do so?

Before you say yes, there are several questions you should ask. What links to and from that site have been authorized? What else is on that site? Who uses that site, and what is its purpose? Who controls the site and could make changes to your work? What if you change your mind and want to remove your work from the site? Is there advertising on the site? Will readers be able to contact you (electronically, or via phone, fax, or mail)? Will that site control the copyright to your material? Does a prior appearance on the Web constitute a prior publication that would prohibit you from submitting the manuscript to a "real" journal?

If you do agree to submit your material, visit the site every now and then, especially if you start getting strange e-mail. If you cannot figure out how someone found your article, it is perfectly legitimate to ask. If you discover that some unsavory or undesirable links are involved, contact the person responsible for maintaining the site that contains your article and request that your material be removed.

Some scientific fields have a system in which nearly all important (and many not-so-important) papers are posted on a Web site before they are peer reviewed and published. This allows instant communication of ideas and results in the field. The main problem with this approach is the lack of quality control. Another is that the newsworthiness and uniqueness of the journal will be diminished if everyone can get access to the information in an article months before it is published.

CONCLUSION

Information on most medical references is instantly available in an electronic format that includes author name(s), title, journal, year, volume, page range, and key words, in online databases such as MEDLINE. The abstracts of many original and review articles are also available electronically; sometimes the full text of an article is provided. An investigator can easily obtain a list of potentially relevant references by searching one of these databases. This remarkable capability can be exploited best if you are adept at doing efficient and thorough searches. Spend an afternoon learning this skill from a professional, such as a medical librarian, or from a published guidebook.[1,2] It will be time well spent, particularly if you work one on one with a librarian doing a "real search" in the area that you are studying. It is a lot easier to learn the ins and outs of searching if you actually care about what you are finding. A general class on "Entrez PubMed" will be better than nothing but not as good as focusing on your own area.

Most investigators locate more than enough references. That is why the ability to separate the wheat from the chaff—to become a critical reader of the literature—is worth developing. You can sharpen this skill by attending journal clubs and reading letters to the editor about articles you have seen. How many of the points that were raised had you previously thought of yourself? Do you agree with these points? Do you think the authors of the original article responded adequately?

Finally, not everything worthwhile was written in the last 3 to 5 years. Be sure to look further back in your literature searches. The basic tools of clinical research—careful observation and analysis—have not changed since 2000, or even since 1900.

CHECKLIST FOR

REFERENCES AND ELECTRONIC PUBLISHING

1. Do you provide a citation for all nonobvious statements of fact, emphasizing reviews and seminal articles?

2. Have you read all cited references to ensure they support the point you made?

3. Has the reference list been updated at the time of manuscript submission and checked for typographical errors?

4. If a manuscript or presentation has been posted on the Web, have you checked the Web site periodically to make sure you are comfortable that it belongs there?

References

1. Stave C. *Field Guide to Medline: Making Searching Simple*. Philadelphia, PA: Lippincott Williams & Wilkins; 2003.
2. Katcher B. *MEDLINE: A Guide to Effective Searching in PubMed and Other Interfaces*. San Francisco, CA: Ashbury Press; 2006.

10 Authorship

Authors are members of the research team who make intellectual contributions to the project, participate in writing the manuscript, review and approve the final version of the manuscript, and are willing to take public responsibility for it. Because disagreements over authorship are common, learning these requirements for authorship will serve you well in your investigative career.

Some of the requirements of authorship—such as review and approve the final version—are easier to define than others. The lead author of the manuscript is responsible for ensuring that all other authors review and approve the final version. Most journals require an article's authors to sign a written statement verifying their willingness to accept responsibility for their article's contents. Only if the manuscript is eventually challenged as fraudulent will "public responsibility" come back to haunt someone who did not participate fully enough in the research to be aware of the fraud. Although every author cannot vouch for every detail in a multiauthor study, all should be sufficiently familiar with the research project and their colleagues to be confident that the results are valid. If that familiarity is lacking, they should not agree to be authors.

Authorship can take many forms, from writing the drafts to revising a particular section, to penciling in extensive changes or suggestions for improvement. Whether someone on the research team who glances at a manuscript, says it looks fine, and makes only a minor comment or two (or none at all) qualifies as an author is less certain. If that person meets all the other requirements and was not given the opportunity to participate in the writing of the manuscript until it was nearly ready for publication, it may not be realistic to expect extensive suggestions or to make them a condition for authorship. If you send a colleague a near-final draft, you are also sending an unwritten message that extensive comments are not welcome. Therefore, it is best to involve potential authors early in the drafting of a manuscript and give them an opportunity to participate. If they choose not to, or do not ever respond, then it is easier to exclude them from the author list.

Perhaps the most difficult requirement of authorship to define is *intellectual contribution*. An individual makes an intellectual contribution when that person participates materially in the project's science by doing at least one of the following:

1. *Formulation of the research question and design of the study.* This does not necessarily mean that all investigators who were present at the study's creation are automatically authors. They need to have been active participants in the scientific development of the study.

2. *Development of critical methodology.* The key word is *critical.* Someone who suggested a change in the wording of a questionnaire or that glucose levels be measured in fasting samples did not make a critical contribution.

3. *Planning the analysis or presentation of the data.* Specific ideas ("We should analyze the data after adjusting for income"; "We should categorize vitamin C intake by milligram per day"; "We should present the results stratified by disease severity") are necessary. Vague suggestions ("You should write up these results") do not suffice.

Not every author's intellectual contribution will be identical, or even comparable, in importance. But all must meet the minimum standard.

If there was no intellectual contribution, there is no authorship. People who just did what they were told—no matter how well they did it—do not meet the requirements for authorship. Activities such as recruiting patients, checking a questionnaire for typographic errors, collecting data, preparing tables under your direction, and finding references in the library do not meet the criteria. This *caveat* can be a problem when a research team has research assistants or technicians who are essential to a study but have not made intellectual contributions. Try to anticipate this problem and clarify the requirements for authorship with team members. Tell them about your research plans and ask them if they have any suggestions. As a junior investigator, you will earn well-deserved kudos if you involve longtime staff members, summer students, or foreign medical graduates looking to enhance their CVs in the intellectual development of a study or manuscript. That way they can earn an authorship role, and you will benefit from their experience and energy. It is also much easier to ask for extra help on short notice from people who see themselves as collaborators and potential authors on a project than it is to ask employees.

I recognize that authorship requirements are more difficult to apply in the real world than they are to talk about abstractly. Some examples may help clarify the distinction between authors and nonauthors (Table 10.1). The phrase, "possibly an author," indicates that a potential author still needs to meet the other requirements. Someone who is "not automatically an author" may qualify by contributing in other ways.

TABLE 10.1	Example of Authors and Nonauthors
Possibly an Author	**Not Automatically an Author**
The director of a clinical center who recruited a few patients for a multicenter study and helped design the sampling scheme and plan for follow-up	The director of the clinical center who recruits the most patients for a multicenter study
A graduate student who interviewed some of the subjects, and who wrote and validated several of the questions	A graduate student who interviewed all the subjects
An investigator who helped develop a new method of measuring substance Y	An investigator in the laboratory next door who let you use his "X machine" to measure substance Y
The statistical analyst who recommended one of several alternate ways to analyze the data	The statistical analyst who analyzed the data following your specific directions
The senior colleague who read the manuscript and rewrote a paragraph or two	The senior colleague who read the manuscript and found a few typos
The head of a laboratory who said that someone should look into this problem, did not provide you with any resources, but met with you periodically to review your work and suggested or approved your approaches	The head of a laboratory who said that someone should look into this problem, furnished you with a bench and a technician, but then did not participate further in the research

Authorship has become something of a *cause célèbre* among journal editors—in part because of concerns that author lists have gotten so long that accountability for articles has, in many instances, become diffused. Another problem is that manuscripts with many authors make it difficult to tell who deserves academic credit for the work. Some academic institutions are dealing with this problem in the promotion process by asking faculty to specify their exact contributions to each manuscript. Under such a system, the value of being the 8th or 10th author is often close to nothing; perhaps in this way the inflation of author lists will eventually cease.

THE PRACTICALITIES

Because it is far easier to add an author than to subtract one, by far the most important advice in this chapter is simple: Start the author list on the first draft of the manuscript or abstract as "Paul Stein (assuming that is your name) and others." Add others *after* they meet the requirements of intellectual contribution and participation in the writing of the manuscript. Once the process is under way, you can politely let would-be authors know that they were too late: "I'm sorry, but the author list is already set. I'd be happy to work with you on my next project. Next time, let's try to arrange something a little sooner."

When in doubt about whether to include a senior colleague, ask if he or she is interested in *helping* with the manuscript. (Do not ask if that colleague is interested in *being* an author.) Make it clear that this role will involve more than just a brief note that says, "Looks great. By the way, I'm now a full professor; please change my title." Spell out the requirements:

> I am calling about the manuscript on the effect of *Helicobacter* on claudication that I am writing. I am asking all of the potential coauthors to do the following. ... In addition, I would like you to pay careful attention to the discussion section. I could use some help with the paragraphs on strengths and limitations of the study. Have I cited the most important articles? Furthermore, did I describe the recruitment process accurately?

Offer a graceful exit in case a colleague is not interested:

> I will understand if you are too busy. Perhaps you would prefer to be recognized in the acknowledgments.

If you do receive an indication of interest, respond with enthusiasm and some specific tasks:

> That is great. I need to have your ideas (comments) (by 3 to 4 weeks from now) to include them in the analysis plan (or presentation manuscript). If I have not heard from you by then, I will assume that it has just turned out that you are too busy.

Note the use of the passive voice, to lay blame on the mysterious time consumers with which all senior investigators seem to feel plagued.

What about adding a senior author to improve the chances of publication? Avoid doing this if it is just for show. Instead, you can say to the journal editors (if such is the case) that "Dr. Well-Known suggested that I submit this article for your consideration." While most editors will insist that they are not influenced by cover letters or name-dropping, human nature argues otherwise.

HOW DOES ONE TELL NONAUTHORS THEIR FATE?

The best way of letting someone know that he or she will not be listed as an author resembles the method party givers use to deal with rowdy guests: Do not invite them in the first place. Never add people to your abstract or title page until they have earned authorship. It may be tempting, especially to junior investigators, to add a more senior person's name to a paper in the hope that he or she will spend more time looking at it. This rarely works. More often than not, unless you are working on a large and obviously important project, you will be fortunate if even one other person is willing to spend a substantial amount of time on your manuscript.

Be alert for freeloaders who make last-minute requests to be listed as authors, especially if you have an important finding. This practice is surprisingly common, sometimes happening even after a manuscript has been accepted, particularly if it is to appear in a prestigious journal. Do not let yourself be forced into adding authors because you were caught unprepared. A colleague may casually suggest, "Go ahead and add me to that manuscript." In most cases, a quick response of, "Gee, I am sorry, but the manuscript is already written and the author list is already set," is all that is needed.

It is harder to turn down a request for authorship when it comes from a senior colleague or department chair whom you do not want to antagonize. It is tempting to advise responding with something like "I did not realize that you had worked on this manuscript," or "I am not sure I feel comfortable having you be responsible for this work," but neither choice is very practical. A better response is flattery, delay, and consultation: "I am flattered that you want to be included. I would like a chance to discuss your request with the other authors." Then seek help from the other authors. Explain the specific problems ("Dr. Uninvolved wants to be an author, but he has not made any contributions to the project."). Ask your other authors for assistance in informing the nonauthor that he does not meet the requirements for authorship.

If none of these suggestions is feasible, then inform potential authors who are really nonauthors that you are planning to submit the manuscript to a particular journal. In reviewing that journal's requirements for authorship, you have determined that only Elise and Michael seem to meet the requirements and that others will be mentioned in the acknowledgments:

> I am afraid the journal insists that all the authors meet a fairly stringent list of requirements. I feel very awkward asking you to sign a statement that is not true. Instead, I would like your permission to thank you for your help in the acknowledgments.

However, do not jeopardize your career over this problem. Sometimes it is a close call as to whether a "want-to-be" author meets the requirements and therefore awkward or impossible to say that you have decided not to include him. In that situation, say yes while insisting that the new coauthor participate in writing the manuscript. Include a time deadline:

> I appreciate your interest in contributing to the manuscript, although I'm afraid that all suggestions must be in by the end of the week. I know that is not very much time. If you do not think you will be able to make substantive suggestions by then, please let me know so I can change the author list. I am sure you realize that it will be awkward for me to bother you about this, and we do want to submit the manuscript expeditiously.

A troubling phenomenon is that of ghost authorship, in which a manuscript is written for the first author by a "hired gun," who may work for the sponsor of the research, such as a pharmaceutical company. The ghost author may be included somewhere in the middle of the author list or may not appear at all. The company may rationalize this behavior because it ensures that certain minimum standards are met. The problem, of course, is that the sponsor's objectives are hardly disinterested. This practice is fundamentally dishonest. While it may be an easy way to add an article to your bibliography that lists you as lead author, in the long run your scientific reputation will be harmed.

ORDER OF AUTHORSHIP

It is usually easiest to determine the first and last authors. The first author writes the drafts of the manuscript. For junior investigators, this usually means that the electronic copy is in the first author's computer. Only in rare circumstances should this principle be violated, such as if someone was responsible for most of the work but subsequently was unable to write the manuscript because of illness or language problems.

If an established research group produced the manuscript, the last-listed author is usually the senior mentor for the group. This assumes that he or she meets the requirements for authorship. This listing is not for a figurehead who just provided laboratory space or access to a database.

The other authors are listed in order of their intellectual contribution to the project. They should not be ranked based on who recruited the most patients (although this is commonly done when ghost authors write articles for pharmaceutical companies) or who spent the most hours in the laboratory. The first author, perhaps in consultation with the senior (last) author, should decide.

Sometimes, a group of authors make essentially equal contributions. Most journals will allow a footnote so indicating or indicating that authors are listed alphabetically. For some large studies, a corporate authorship is provided. If you are a junior investigator who is fortunate enough to be the lead author on such a project, try to be cited by name (e.g., Rosenthal D for the Mega-Trial Investigators' Group) to enhance recognition of your name.

HOW AND WHEN DO YOU MOVE YOURSELF UP OR DOWN ON THE LIST?

There will be times when you functioned as the first or second author on a manuscript but have been listed lower on the list. Speak to the first author or senior author. Spell out your concerns:

> I am now the fifth author, but I think I have done more work than everyone else but you. I prepared three of the tables and rewrote the methods section.

> I am listed as second author, but I have been acting as the first author. I have written everything but one of the tables and the subjects section. I have taken responsibility for moving the project forward, although it was originally assigned to Linda.

Make your suggestions, anticipate concerns, and offer solutions:

> I would like to be second author. I would be happy to talk with Marilyn and Mel about this.

> I think I should be first author. I realize this was supposed to be Sylvia's project, but I think it is better for the project if we go forward with me in the lead.

Be prepared for a pleasant surprise. Most people respond quite reasonably. Many are even relieved that someone else is willing to step forward to resuscitate what might well be a dying manuscript. But if you meet resistance, do not bristle. Suggest deferring the decision until you both have had time to talk it over with colleagues. Offer to schedule a meeting of all the authors to make a decision.

Order of authorship can become more of an issue if one of the authors suffers from tenure and promotion anxiety. A previously delightful colleague may change his stripes when being evaluated for promotion. He suddenly realizes that he is an article or two short, or that being first author matters. Try gently pointing out the problem: "I can understand your desire to be first author, given your upcoming evaluation for tenure. But I am sure you agree that this has been my project from the beginning and that you can understand that being first author is important to me also." If that fails, seek help from a senior colleague on the project or in your department.

Another problem can arise when a first author is unable or unwilling to write a manuscript but will not relinquish first-authorship rights. This situation can persist for months or years, as a series of excuses are provided. Eventually, the coauthors realize that something needs to be done, but no one wants to take responsibility for reassigning the manuscript. If you find yourself in this situation—as a coauthor who is willing to serve as first author of a stalled manuscript—then the best approach is to be straightforward. Talk with the senior author, if there is one, and ask that he or she reassign the manuscript. If there is no senior author, then contact the current first author to see if he or she has any objections to your plan to contact the other investigators with a brief note such as the following:

> Due to her increasingly busy clinical workload, Elin has been unable to work on the manuscript for the past 18 months. In the interest of moving the project forward, I will be willing to take responsibility for serving as first author and producing a first draft within the next 60 days. Elin and I have discussed this option, and it is mutually agreeable. Please contact me if you have any questions.

WHAT CONSTITUTES A PAPER?

Defining what constitutes a paper is another authorship issue, but in a bit of disguise. The problem may emerge when a research group has divided a project into several parts, so that several different investigators can each be first author of a manuscript. It may also manifest itself because a 500-word summary of the project was previously published in the proceedings of a meeting.

Original research that has already been presented at a meeting can almost always be submitted in manuscript form. This includes abstracts, posters, and oral presentations. Such may not be the case, however, for extensive reports in conference proceedings; check with the journal editor by sending a copy of the report with the manuscript.

However, just because you have different first authors does not mean you have different manuscripts. Consider, for example, a study involving the use of ultrasound in making a diagnosis of renal stones. Is it acceptable to present the same results in separate journals aimed at emergency physicians, radiologists, urologists, and family practitioners? Unfortunately, the answer is no, and most journals require authors to indicate that the work has not been submitted elsewhere. Editors take this very seriously. They see themselves as protectors of the integrity of the scientific literature. While it may not seem like a big deal to you or your coauthors to simultaneously submit a different version of the manuscript to a completely unrelated journal, it is extremely important to them. You do not want to be accused of duplicate publication, so make that sure you are the only one in your research group who is submitting a manuscript based on a single set of results.

It can sometimes be difficult to tell whether a group of findings constitutes one paper or two. First of all, are the data insufficient for even one paper? Because these issues can be difficult for a new author to resolve, you should seek advice from experienced colleagues, if possible. If you cannot, there are several clues that a project is too big for a single manuscript. For example, when you sit down to write the manuscript, if you find that you have several research questions, or more than five or six key points, then you may have more than one manuscript (especially if those key points are unrelated). If the manuscript is never finished and each revision seems to travel in a new direction, you probably have more than one manuscript. In some instances, a single large study may be the seedbed for dozens of unique manuscripts, all of them based on the same subjects and measurements. If each addresses a unique research question, then each may warrant a separate manuscript.

There are times when yet another manuscript from the same study is not needed. If you find yourself repeating the same Methods section several times in different manuscripts, that should raise a red flag that perhaps multiple publications are not warranted. Having only one paragraph of new results is another clue that you do not have another complete manuscript.

Sometimes the best option is not another full-length original article but a letter to the editor or a brief report. If you have made an important observation, subsequent investigators who cite your study will not be concerned about the length of your manuscript.

When in doubt about whether a manuscript warrants a separate publication, mention other manuscripts from the same study in a cover letter to the editors. Cite the references if the studies are published or include a copy of the abstract of any unpublished manuscripts. Some journals may want copies of the complete manuscripts, so be prepared to adhere to such a request. In your letter, indicate how the current manuscript differs from those from your group that have been previously published or submitted.

ACKNOWLEDGMENTS

A brief acknowledgment at the end of a manuscript is another way to express appreciation to people who worked on the project. This is particularly appropriate for someone who put in extra effort but did not meet the criteria for authorship. A colleague who referred patients for study, allowed you to borrow some materials, or read the drafts of the manuscript might fall into this category. These small acknowledgements are often very meaningful, particularly to someone who has never seen their name in print in a scientific journal.

Some journals require written permission to acknowledge someone. Persons who are acknowledged must agree to be named and to have their contribution listed.

A SPECIAL PLEA TO SENIOR INVESTIGATORS

Resist the temptation to pad your bibliography by forcing your name onto an author list when you do not belong. You do not get to be an author just because you paid someone's salary, signed a visa request, lent a computer or a technician, allowed access to your database or fancy machine, or were selected as the department chair. It is almost impossible for your junior colleagues to decline an inappropriate request from you for author status; do not put them in that position. If you feel compelled to be included in every manuscript that your department or research group produces, then earn that privilege by mentoring junior colleagues and meeting the requirements for authorship.

(Junior investigators—if appropriate, make a copy of the paragraph above and leave it anonymously in a senior colleague's mailbox. It may not help matters, but you will probably feel a little better.)

CONCLUSION

Like being an investigator, being the author of a manuscript is a privilege. Make sure that when your name appears on a manuscript you have earned that privilege and the manuscript is one in which you take pride.

CHECKLIST FOR
AUTHORSHIP

1. Does everyone included as an author meet the requirements for authorship?

2. Has anyone who deserves to be an author been left out?

3. Have all authors reviewed and approved the final version of the manuscript submitted?

4. Does the order of authorship correlate with contributions made to the manuscript, with the possible exception of the last author?

11

Posters

If it is the first time you have submitted an abstract to a meeting, you will likely be thrilled to learn that your work has been accepted as a poster presentation. But what exactly will that involve? What will you need to do between the time that your abstract has been accepted and the time to display your poster?

For those of you who have never attended a scientific meeting, poster sessions are a bit like science fairs without the doting parents. You will be expected to prepare a summary of your work, post it on a bulletin board in a large room, and stand next to it for a few hours while discussing your work with passersby.

Preparing a poster will take longer than you think. As the time draws closer, you will realize that standing beside a poorly done piece of work for 2 or 3 hours will not be much fun. You will want your poster to reflect the quality of your research. So unless you are one of those people who does not embarrass easily, plan on spending at least a full day preparing your poster, not including the time it takes to assemble and analyze your data.

In some instances, posters are displayed for the duration of the meeting, with designated hours when the authors are supposed to be available. At other meetings, posters are displayed for a limited time, then replaced by the next group. Sometimes poster sessions are well attended and become a valuable experience for the poster presenters. At other meetings, the posters are largely ignored; for those meetings, experienced investigators may choose the "oral presentation only" box on the abstract submission form to avoid having to prepare a poster that will go unnoticed. Ask colleagues who have attended the meeting in previous years how posters are usually received.

THE BASICS

If your abstract is accepted as a poster, the meeting organizers will send you guidance on the poster session. This includes the times your poster needs to be set up and taken down, and the time you are expected to be in attendance. The instructions will also tell you how big the poster should be as well as specific details about format. Pay careful attention to the information on the maximum size of your poster. If the poster is too big, there will be no alternative to watching it flop around, in constant danger of being bent by errant visitors. Some of the other details are usually less essential. For example, the meeting sponsors will not make you remove your poster if the title letters are only 8 cm instead of 10 cm high. However, most of the suggestions are made for your benefit, so that viewers will be able to read your poster from the usual viewing distance of a few feet.

Before beginning to prepare your poster, you must decide whether it will have a single panel or multiple panels. A single-panel poster consists of one large sheet of paper on which the entire poster is printed (Fig. 11-1). You then simply pin the entire poster in place. Single-panel posters are usually done professionally and look terrific, but they are expensive to make. The exact price will depend on how much "editing" needs to be done before the poster can be printed, the use of color, the type of paper, and, most important, how quickly you need to have the poster made. Sometimes the number of figures and photographs affects the cost.

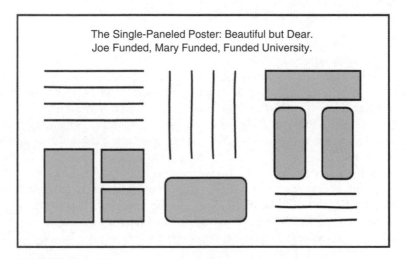

The Single-Paneled Poster: Beautiful but Dear.
Joe Funded, Mary Funded, Funded University.

FIGURE 11-1. The single-panel poster

Many companies will print a full-size poster from a file that you have made using desktop publishing or presentation software. If you cannot create your own poster for someone else to print, there are even companies that can do the layout for your poster from your rough design and data. But be warned—having your poster made professionally does not absolve you from the task of preparing it. You still have to tell the poster maker what to include. You need to be especially sure that there are no errors in the material because once the poster has been made, corrections are expensive.

Although few investigators these days make multipanel posters, it does not mean that you should rule out that option, particularly if you are running late and the alternative is to not have any poster at all.

GETTING STARTED

Begin with a sketch of the overall design of your poster. An ordinary piece of paper, turned on its side, will represent the usual shape of most posters. Read the instructions to be sure. Every now and then a poster session is held in a room with strangely shaped bulletin boards.

Draw a large banner across the top for the title, and several (no more than 10) boxes for the panels or sections. Usually, as shown in Figure 11-2, panels are ordered from top left to bottom right, in vertical columns; numbering each panel (in the right-hand corner) helps the reader get oriented.

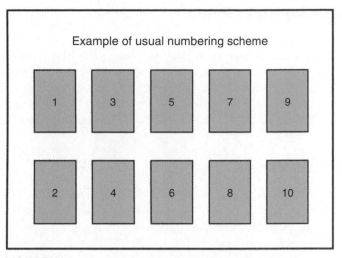

FIGURE 11-2. The usual order of panels in a poster

GENERAL ADVICE ABOUT PANELS OR COMPONENTS OF THE POSTER

Do not plan on including the abstract itself unless required. Abstracts are usually dense and hard to read, and they should already be available in the meeting's proceedings.

As a general rule for font sizes, the title of the poster should be about 85 point; authors' names, 56 point; sub-headers, 36 point; text, 24 point; and legends and captions, 18 point.

Use left-justified text only (or center justified for titles). Do not both right- and left-justify. Use both upper- and lowercase letters, as they are easier to read. If you use a sans serif font (e.g., Arial, Helvetica, Univers, or Verdana) for the text and titles, then use a serif-based font (e.g., Garamond, Palatino, or Times) for the figure legends and tables, or vice versa. Do not use more than two fonts (one for text, one for tables, etc.) in your poster.

Give legibility priority over details. There is no need to use complete sentences when describing methods and results, but they are helpful in the background and conclusions sections. Use boldface type, bullets and arrows, and boxes to emphasize important points. Use underlining and italics sparingly.

Most panels (or parts of the poster) should have a brief title, such as *Subjects* or *Limitations*. A title may not be needed for the first panel if it begins with an engaging question. Keep the titles of the panels simple so that they fit in a line or two.

The top row of your poster (the odd-numbered panels in Fig. 11-2) are always easier to see than the bottom row. So, if at all possible, put your most important information (background, main results, and conclusions) in the top row, even if it means that not every panel is in exactly the right order. For example, you may have to put your conclusions in position 9 and the study's limitations in position 10.

What follows is a brief summary of what belongs to each panel. More details on content can be found in the specific chapters dealing with the different sections of the research paper.

Introduction/Background Panel

If your title is particularly on the dry side, it helps to have some text that catches the attention of the casual observer in the first panel. This should be a few sentences long or perhaps be in the form of a brief question. It should be printed in relatively large, bold type. Be creative, even controversial. The remainder of the background panel should include enough information about your study to enable the reader to understand why you did it. Rarely should this section occupy more than one panel.

Subjects/Methods Panels

Plan on having two to four panels for your Methods, although you may be able to fit all of the relevant details on a single panel. Provide the basic details about the study design, subjects, measurements, and analysis methods, and provide more details about any unique methods you used.

Results Panels

Usually, you will have three to five panels of results. Whether you use tables or figures to convey your main results, it is important to explain what is in them in the title. It should be possible for a visitor who takes the time to look at your poster to remember what you found. The title of each panel should tell the reader what the results in the panel show: "Life Is Tough for Junior Faculty," "Life Is Even Tougher for Junior Faculty with Small Children," and "Life Is Toughest of All for Junior Faculty with Small Children and a Working Spouse." Do not simply label your panels "Results of First Analysis."

Limitations Panel

Include the main limitations of your study, whether they relate to the small number of subjects, missing data, the less-than-perfect design, or the imprecision of some of your measurements.

Conclusions and Implications Panel

Do not just repeat the results; explain them. Make your best guess as to what they mean. Indicate specific directions for your next projects. Make clinical and scientific recommendations, if appropriate.

 ## EXAMPLE POSTER

The following example provides the content found in a typical poster.

PANEL 1

Background

- We previously found an association between low bone density and mortality in elderly women.

- Hormone levels and renal function change with age.
- Renal function has been associated with bone density.

PANEL 2

Research Questions

- Is there an association between hormones involved in bone metabolism and mortality?
- Is there an association between renal function and mortality?
- Is there an association between renal function and bone mineral density?

PANEL 3

Methods

- Study of Osteoporotic Fractures
- Prospective cohort of 9,704 white women (age 65 years)
- Questionnaire, interview, weight, bone density at baseline
- Serum samples, stored at −190°C
- Mean follow-up of 6.7 years
- Case–cohort method
  - 90 randomly selected deaths
  - 396 randomly selected controls, 56 of whom died
- Cause of death from death certificates, hospital records
  - Cardiovascular = 54
  - Cancer = 58
- Blindly measured hormones, creatinine; stability verified
- Creatinine clearance estimated as:

  (140 − age in years) × weight in kg (72 × Cr in mg/dL)

  Analysis with proportional hazards models

PANEL 4

Mortality Declines with Higher Creatinine Clearance

- Mortality was 62% (95% CI: 25% to 81%) lower in women with estimated clearance >73 mL/minute than in those with clearances <50 mL/minute. Excluding the three women with serum creatinine values >2.0 mg/dL (18 mmol/L) did not affect results.

PANEL 5

Limitations

- Elderly white women only.
- Number of deaths owing to specific causes was small.
- Measurement of creatinine was made only once. Cystatin C was not measured.
- Cockcroft–Gault equation estimates creatinine clearance, thereby *underestimating the* magnitude of association between actual renal function and mortality.

PANEL 6

Why Is Renal Function Associated with Mortality?

- Renal function as a marker for underlying disease? Adjustment for diabetes, hypertension had no effect.
- Nonspecific manifestation of poor health? Adjustment for albumin had no effect.
- Direct effect of reduction in clearance? Only one death was because of renal failure.
- Impaired ability to respond to other medical problems?

Implications

- Measure renal function in epidemiologic studies of mortality in the elderly.
- Preservation of renal function may be associated with reduced mortality.

USING PRESENTATION SOFTWARE TO MAKE A SINGLE-PANEL POSTER

After assembling the components of your poster, the next steps are to insert those parts into a single file (most likely a PowerPoint document) to be printed professionally. Get a template for your poster, either from colleagues or from the media office at your institution—or even from another institution's Web site. (I am not suggesting plagiarism of content, just borrowing the format.) Starting from a template is infinitely easier that trying to create one from scratch. Determine the maximum size of the poster from the information provided by the meeting organizers. Use the "Page Setup" menu in the Design tab, with the slides sized for "Custom" in the pull-down menu, and enter the dimensions of the poster. Make sure they are in inches or cm, as appropriate; also check that you have not inadvertently switched the horizontal and vertical dimensions. You do not have to use the entire allotted space; indeed, it is a good idea to make your poster 4 or 5 cm smaller than the maximum allowed.

After the individual "components" (e.g., background, methods, figures, etc.) are perfect, add them to the template. Convert images to JPEG files, and use the Insert command—do not just cut and paste. Add your institution's logo, if appropriate.

If you are importing photographic images, be very careful about touching them up. As a rule, overall changes (e.g., in color and sharpness) are less likely to compromise scientific integrity than local changes to a particular region of the image. Most of the time, you will need professional help to scan nondigital images, such as 35-mm slides and radiographs. If you scan a photograph yourself, do not forget to clean the scanner glass.

Check for mistakes by spell checking and by printing a copy of the poster on plain paper.

The PowerPoint file can then be e-mailed to the graphics design office at your institution or to one of the many companies that print posters (search the Web for "scientific poster printing") and send them back to you in handy tubes. You will pay more, often much more, for rush jobs, so plan ahead. You will also pay more if you send in the components and have the printer assemble them into a poster. But this is sometimes a good option, especially if you have several posters to make and only two hands and 4 hours available to you. If you are running especially late, ask the printing company to express ship the poster directly to the hotel at which you are staying.

MAKING A MULTIPLE-PANEL POSTER

If you are making a multiple-panel poster (Fig. 11-3), you can wait until almost the last minute to prepare it because you can print the individual panels yourself on a laser printer. If you bring a portable computer, you can even make last-minute changes by sending a revised version of a panel to your hotel's fax machine or printing a copy in the business office. Prepare your poster on several sheets of paper, which you can mount on sheets of colored paper or cardboard (say, red or blue). Cardboard is better because it will not bend as easily in transport. A multiple-panel poster will not look nearly as professional as a single-panel version, but it may convey the message (intended or not) that you were so busy as an investigator that you did not have time to prepare a professional-style poster!

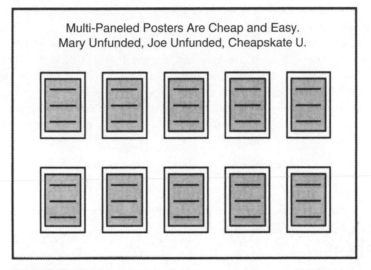

FIGURE 11-3. The multiple-panel poster

Even if you are making the panels yourself, have the banner (the section of the poster listing the title and authors) made professionally, sized to fit. A title that has been patched together from several sheets of ordinary-sized paper looks tacky. Fortunately, you will know the title and authors long before you have to prepare the poster itself. If you are planning on making the multiple-panel poster yourself, place an order to have the banner made to the required specifications the day you receive your acceptance notice.

GETTING THE MOST OUT OF A POSTER SESSION

Act like the host at a party. When guests arrive, greet them. Read their name badges and introduce yourself and your friend, "the poster." Practice saying, "Would you like me to take you through the poster? The main points I would like to emphasize are...."

Meet your neighbors. Chat with them if no one else is around. You are looking for potential collaborators and future reviewers of your work. Think of 5 or 10 investigators in your field whom you want to meet and who seem likely to attend the meeting. Look for invited guests or session chairs in the program. Decide what you might say to each of them. If you spot someone you would like to meet, even if that person appears to be passing your poster by, stick out your hand and say "Hello, Dr. Famous. I read your recent study in the *Juneau Journal of Genetics*, and I am pleased to meet you. I am Alice Not-yet-famous, and I work with Dr. Khotani in San Francisco." It is very unlikely that Dr. Famous will bite.

When someone does come by to express interest in your work, do not assume that he or she wants a 10-minute spiel. Plan on spending no more than 2 minutes explaining what you have found. Practice that 2-minute spiel covering the three or four most important points that you want to make. Pay attention to clues from your visitors—if they want more information, they will ask for it. It is much better to respond to specific questions than to lecture. When they start looking away or checking their abstract book, take the hint and thank them for stopping by. Do not forget to ask interested visitors what they are working on—it is a great way to find potential collaborators and contacts.

Do not take it personally if almost no one drops in. Most poster viewers are impulse shoppers. Your topic may not interest them. Although it is awfully boring to stand at an unloved poster and hope that someone will stop by, there are many worse jobs in the world. So do not abandon your poster; host it during the specified hours. Almost always, a few attendees will be interested. They are the organized ones who may have a list of posters to visit, and they may not get to yours until late in the session. Hang in there.

CHECKLIST FOR
POSTERS

1. Does the poster include the basic elements (Introduction, Methods, Results, Limitations, and Conclusions)?

2. Are the main results easy to spot?

3. Have you prepared a short talk about your findings?

4. Have you planned how you will greet people who visit your poster?

12

Oral Presentations

Your ability to present information orally will have a major impact on your scientific career. With few exceptions, investigators who speak well appear more professional and knowledgeable, and their work seems more interesting. Fortunately, almost anyone can learn how to communicate information to an audience effectively.

One speaker I know and enjoy has a style that can best be labeled "locomotive." She pushes ahead at a relentless pace and probably would not even stop for a major earthquake. Her talks are entirely serious, without a hint of humor. But she marshals her arguments clearly and logically, and the audience sits in rapt attention.

Other speakers are more informal. They stroll to the front of the podium, make eye contact with the audience, and offer funny anecdotes. Again, the audience is actively engaged. Both these speaking styles, and many others, work well.

The most important rule is simple—know your audience. If you can anticipate its expectations, then you at least have a chance of meeting them. Expectations commonly concern the format of your talk (e.g., 10 minutes with slides and 5 minutes for questions), its substance (your study), and its style. If the audience expects you to wear a suit and to present the facts and just the facts without any *New Yorker* cartoons, then do so.

Try to provide something interesting for your listeners, perhaps a sentence or two of historical background, an anecdote from a study participant, or even a mistake that you made along the way. If you have ever attended scientific meetings, you know how interminable they can seem. Attendees may hear 20 or 30 presentations in a day, and some meetings go on for a week. Give the audience something to remember about you and your study—after all, that is why you worked so hard to be selected for an oral presentation in the first place.

THE BASIC ORDER OF A PRESENTATION

The order of presentation for a speech is the same as for a manuscript. Begin with a title slide that includes the name of your study and the list of authors and their institutions. Assuming the number of authors is reasonable (if it is not, see Chapter 10), you will even have room at the bottom of the slide for special thanks, if appropriate. Here is an example of a Title slide:

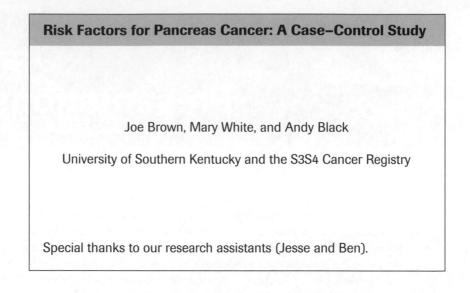

Some investigators feel obliged to begin a talk by acknowledging their coinvestigators and announcing all of their names to the audience. This is a surefire way to start your presentation on the wrong foot. It is dull to listen to someone read a list of names. Doing so implies to the audience that all you are going to do is read your slides, so they have your permission to stop listening. You might as well just flip through your slides without saying anything; at least that way you will stand out!

Instead, while your title slide is visible, thank the chair of the session. Then look the audience in the eye while saying something like, "This morning I would like to present the results of our study on risk factors for lumbago in kangaroos living in North American zoos." Speak directly and forcefully to the back row of the audience, at least for this one sentence. This introduction tells the audience what to expect; it clears out the cobwebs between their ears, and revs up the relevant synapses. You want the audience to realize that if they pay attention to what you *say*, they may actually learn something that is not on the slides. The audience can read the names of your coauthors (who are also listed in the book of abstracts). If it is appropriate, you may wish to mention one or two coauthors or research associates, particularly if they made a special contribution and are in the audience. Then, click to the next slide.

Background

In the next part of your talk, you need to explain why you did your study. This will take a slide or two. Do not try to save a slide by explaining the background for the study while the title slide is visible. Keep the level of detail to a minimum, but be sure to mention what was "unknown" at the time you started your study.

Use the oral part of the presentation to fill in any missing details that the audience needs to know. Cite a specific study if it is relevant.

Next, you need a slide for your research question, which is a simple statement of what you set out to do in the study (or analysis) that you are about to present. Note that one research project may have several research questions. For example, you and your colleagues may have studied the risk factors for several abdominal cancers as part of a larger project. If you are not going to be presenting results for those other

---

Background

Previous studies have identified risk factors for pancreas cancer

  Alcohol use

  Obesity

  Tobacco

Did not determine the effect of having *all* three of these risk factors

---

cancers, then they are not part of the research question for this particular presentation. However, you should mention something like, "Today I am going to present the results of our analysis of the risk factors for pancreas cancer. These data were gathered as part of a larger project looking at the effects of smoking and alcohol on all gastrointestinal malignancies."

Research Question

To identify whether the combination of several common conditions (smoking, alcohol, and obesity) is associated with a greater-than-expected risk of pancreas cancer.

Methods

Next, tell the audience what you did. It helps if you segue into the Methods section by saying something like, "To answer this question, we enrolled 140 cases of pancreas cancer and a similar number of controls. We measured their consumption of coffee, alcohol, and cigarettes using standard instruments, as well as by review of medical records." The slide can then present information about the sample, how you made the diagnosis of pancreatic cancer, and the methods you used to measure and define the predictor variables. As the audience looks at the slide, mention details that you think they may be wondering about (such as the completeness of the cancer registry in those two states, or whether you confirmed the pathologic diagnoses).

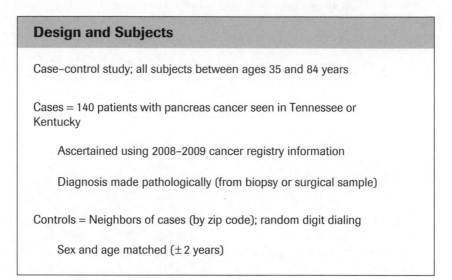

Design and Subjects

Case–control study; all subjects between ages 35 and 84 years

Cases = 140 patients with pancreas cancer seen in Tennessee or Kentucky

    Ascertained using 2008–2009 cancer registry information

    Diagnosis made pathologically (from biopsy or surgical sample)

Controls = Neighbors of cases (by zip code); random digit dialing

    Sex and age matched (± 2 years)

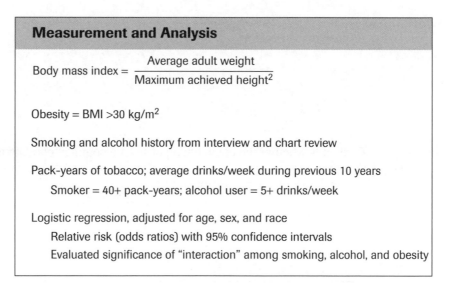

Measurement and Analysis

$$\text{Body mass index} = \frac{\text{Average adult weight}}{\text{Maximum achieved height}^2}$$

Obesity = BMI >30 kg/m^2

Smoking and alcohol history from interview and chart review

Pack-years of tobacco; average drinks/week during previous 10 years
    Smoker = 40+ pack-years; alcohol user = 5+ drinks/week

Logistic regression, adjusted for age, sex, and race
    Relative risk (odds ratios) with 95% confidence intervals
    Evaluated significance of "interaction" among smoking, alcohol, and obesity

The objective is to use spoken and written words together. Rarely is it necessary to read something verbatim from the slide. For example, if you used a tagged radioimmunofluorescent solid-phase assay that was developed by Hendrickson and Klein in 2006, you can put one of those pieces of information (perhaps the one that is hardest to say) on the slide, while you talk about the other.

Most talks also require that you tell about how you analyzed your data. As discussed in Chapter 5, be sure to cover more than just the statistical tests that you used. Also mention how you defined your variables.

Results

Often, you will need to begin this section of your talk by telling the audience a little about the characteristics of your subjects, and, if appropriate, what happened to them during the study. Do not spend too much time on this, however, because what the audience really wants to know is what *answer* you found out to the research question, and listeners will begin to get edgy if you string them along before you get to the "good stuff."

Characteristics of the Subjects		
	Cases (*n* =140)	Controls (*n* =140)
	Percent or mean ± SD	
Age (years)	68.7 ± 9.6	69.3 ± 10.3
Sex (male)	56%	56%
Race (white)	74%	72%
Smoker (40+ pack-years)	39%	26%
Alcohol user (5+ drinks/week)	14%	9%
Body mass index (kg/m^2)	29.3 ± 12.2	27.4 ± 11.6

Again, complement what is on the slide with what you say. For example, if the slide lists the mean ages in the two groups, you might tell the audience the proportion that was over age 65 years. If the slide shows a relative risk of 1.9 when smokers and nonsmokers are compared, then say, "Smoking about doubled the risk of pancreas cancer." If appropriate, say, "All of these results are adjusted for the other variables listed on the slide, as well as age, sex, and race."

Risk Factors for Pancreatic Cancer	
Variable	Relative Risk (95% Confidence Interval)
Smoker	1.9 (1.2–2.9)
Alcohol user	1.3 (0.9–2.0)
Obese	1.5 (0.7–3.3)

But most important, be sure that you present the answer to your research question. In this case, the audience would have been waiting to hear whether the effect of having all three risk factors (smoking, alcohol, and obesity) was greater than expected, so you will certainly need to discuss that particular result, usually with a separate slide. In this case, you would tell the audience (perhaps using the laser pointer as a highlighter), "The P <0.01 indicates that the net effect of having all three risk factors was significantly greater than expected."

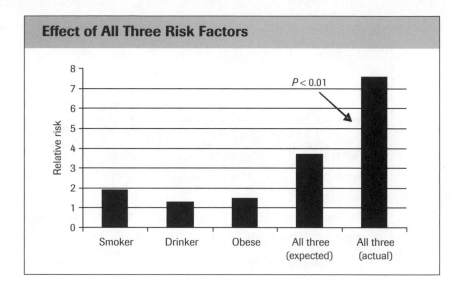

Try to anticipate the audience's questions. In this situation, those hearing your talk would likely want to know the effect of using a different definition of obesity (or of smoking or alcohol use), or of treating body weight, tobacco use, and alcohol consumption as continuous variables. A good presentation provides the answers to questions as those listening to the talk are formulating them.

Similar Results Using Alternate Definitions

Effects of all three risk factors greater than expected (at $P < 0.05$) if...:

   Used different cut points for obesity, smoking, and alcohol use

      BMI > 32 kg/m^2;

      Smoking = 20+pack-years;

      Alcohol = 10+drinks/week

   Treated BMI, tobacco, and alcohol as continuous variables

Finally, if your data have changed substantially since you submitted your abstract, then you need to let the audience know and explain why: "Please note that these results differ from those in the printed abstract. The current results include data from an additional 50 cases."

Limitations

All studies have limitations. You want to indicate that you are aware of them and suggest how you tried to deal with them.

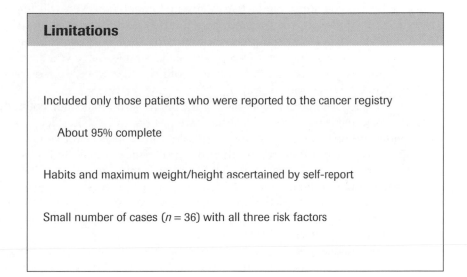

Limitations

Included only those patients who were reported to the cancer registry

About 95% complete

Habits and maximum weight/height ascertained by self-report

Small number of cases ($n = 36$) with all three risk factors

Conclusions and Implications

Try to fit your conclusions onto just a slide or two, emphasizing your main findings. Do not forget to interpret your results for the audience, and discuss any potential implications that your work may have for clinical practice or for understanding the biology of a disease.

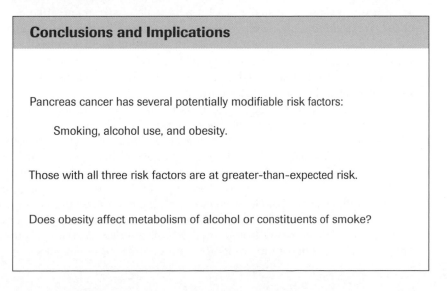

Conclusions and Implications

Pancreas cancer has several potentially modifiable risk factors:

Smoking, alcohol use, and obesity.

Those with all three risk factors are at greater-than-expected risk.

Does obesity affect metabolism of alcohol or constituents of smoke?

Always end your talk by indicating to the audience that you have finished. Do not just run out of slides, or look up aimlessly. Stop for a second or two, regard the audience, say, "Thank you for your attention" and relax.

MAKING YOUR SLIDES

Do not start making your slides until you know what you are going to say. As you get more experienced, you can work directly in PowerPoint or whatever presentation software you are going to use. Many beginners, however, will find it easier to draw 10 or 15 "boxes" on sheets of paper, label them (Title, Background, Methods, etc.) and use that as the template for preparing their talk. Starting out with pencil and paper will also help you to keep your slides simple. Once you have set the basic format and content, you can then transfer your penciled-in version to PowerPoint (or some other presentation software).

Plan on having about one slide per minute of the talk, not counting the title slide. Avoid using transition slides that have just one word ("Results"), as the accompanying oral text ("I'm now going to present the results.") is obvious.

If you are using PowerPoint, then the procedure for making horizontal slides is straightforward, and the size of the slide and its format are preset. If for some reason you are going to prepare your slides using a word processor, and have the printed version photographed, you should aim to produce a version that is 13 cm wide and 8 cm tall. Avoid vertical slides if possible. Some meetings forbid them entirely, as they often do not fit onto the screen.

Find someone in your research group or institution who is a PowerPoint expert (there is always at least one), and have him show you how to use the Master slide to set the background, design, fonts, and so on for your slides.

Avoid using "fancy" templates for your slides. The color schemes are suboptimal for maximum visibility, and extraneous graphic features can be distracting. Choose a simple background without extra doodads. Your institutional logo need not appear on every slide, even if the graphics folks made your slides. A brief appearance on the first slide will suffice.

The simplest slides—black print on a white background, perhaps using blue or red for emphasis—are usually just fine; they also have the advantage that the room need not be kept dark for the slides to be visible. If you do not want to use black on white, consider using a basic blue background, with a yellow title, white text, and one other color (e.g., pink) for bullets or to highlight important results. The blue should be a medium shade (the color of a gas flame); darker tones do not provide enough light if the room is very dark.

If you need to use more colors, as in a figure with several bars, remember that all the colors must contrast with the background and with each other. If you are using a blue background, be aware that thin lines (i.e., in figures) often do not show up very well against it, particularly if the lines are red, green, black, or similar colors. Consider using thick, lighter-colored (e.g., pink, light green, yellow-orange, or even white) lines.

You will almost never need more than five colors. Using diagonal slashes or horizontal lines in the bars is often easier on the audience's eyes than using different colors. Remember that several members of your audience are likely to be unable to distinguish red and green. If you must use those colors as bars in a figure, consider "cross-hatching" one of the colors for your color-blind colleagues.

Warning: Do not rely on the audience's ability to distinguish a thin white line from a thin yellow line, or a thin yellow line from a thin green line. Make sure that the lines are at least 2 points wide, and also use dots and dashes, or connected triangles, squares, and circles, as well as colors to distinguish them. Use the same scheme in each figure and orient your audience to it. If there is a logical reason to use a particular color for a particular group, then do so: "The blue dotted lines represent men; the red solid lines represent women. The lollipop circles indicate subjects with diabetes; the triangles represent subjects without diabetes." Whatever you do, do not change the meaning of those colors or shapes in the middle of a presentation.

Do not animate slides for a scientific presentation. It is distracting for the audience to see information flying on and off the screen; more important, it is easy to forget to hit the "advance" key in the middle of a presentation, particularly when you are nervous. If that happens, you may find yourself losing your train of thought, as what was supposed to be the next slide turns out to be a cute new bullet that pinwheels in slowly with data on a point that you have already made.

SLIDE FORMAT

Your slides serve as reminders to you about what to talk about next, and they give the audience something to look at while listening to you. Keep them as brief as possible. Do not use a sentence when a simple phrase is enough, and do not use a phrase if a word or two suffice.

Use a one-line title for each slide, in a slightly bigger font than the text. There is no need to number the titles of slides (e.g., Methods 1, Methods 2) nor do you need to say, "Methods: Subjects." Just title the slide "Subjects." Use a maximum of seven lines of text. Try to keep each point to a single line.

Tables should have no more than three or four columns and five to seven rows (this does not count the headers for the columns). If you were to multiply the number of rows by the number of columns, the product should be <15 and preferably <10. For example, if your table has four rows, you should have only two or three columns ($4 \times 2 = 8$; $4 \times 3 = 12$).

Slides must be readable from the back of the room. Do not embarrass yourself with a slide that has tiny print and forces you to say, "If you could read this slide, you could see that...."

If you use the same format for several slides (e.g., figures that have the same x and y axes but present results for different groups of subjects), orient the audience the first time, "I am going to be showing you several slides like this, so I want to orient you...." If a slide looks similar, but is not, warn the audience, "Unlike the previous slides, in this slide...."

The principle of orienting the audience also applies to tables. Tell the audience what appears in each column and walk it through one of the rows. If you do not tell the audience what is in a slide, everyone will be too busy trying to figure it out to pay attention to what you are saying.

Avoid footnotes on slides. They are too hard to see. If you must use asterisks for significant P values, tell the audience what they mean.

TIMING YOUR TALK

Time matters. Plan your talk carefully. People get bored and annoyed listening to speakers who are disorganized or sloppy. Once it is obvious that you are running late and have started to rush to make up time, the audience stops paying attention to you, and just wishes you would finish, already. They figure that if you have decided that something is not essential and can be hustled through, then they do not have to pay attention. This is a universal phenomenon, no matter how wonderful your talk. It is much better to have extra time than it is to rush. So aim for a talk that is about 10% shorter than the allotted time.

If you run overtime in your practice sessions (see under "Practicing Your Talk"), consider each section of the talk separately. Can the background be shortened, given the likely familiarity of the audience with the topic? Can you eliminate a detailed description of well-accepted methods? Are your conclusions simply a rehash of what you said two slides previously?

WHAT TO SAY

There are several approaches to preparing the oral materials that will accompany your slides. Whatever you do, do not read your slides. That is what the audience is doing. The easiest way to keep yourself from reading a slide is to follow the rules for making good slides. Doing so will ensure that there are few complete sentences on your slides, and, as a general rule, speaking in complete sentences is a good idea.

Many presenters prefer to have their talk written down, word for word, exactly as they plan to deliver it. This can be dull for listeners. If this is your choice, practice enough so you do not actually have to read the talk. It is also easy to read too quickly. If you have a tendency to speed up when you get anxious, then write, "Slow down. Breathe" in big letters at the bottom of every other page.

If you do write out your talk, print it in at least 14-point type (i.e., 2 points bigger than standard typescript). Often, the lighting at the podium is inadequate, and it can be hard to read smaller fonts. For ease of reading, use double-spaced capital and lowercase letters, rather than all capitals. Do not forget to number the pages and to indicate what text accompanies which slide.

Another technique is to prepare an outline of your talk, with selected key points or phrases for each slide. This ensures that you will not forget to mention a crucial detail, but allows sufficient latitude so that you can make changes in response to previous talks.

As you gain experience, you may prefer to wing it, giving an extemporaneous talk. The main dangers of making this decision are that you may leave out something important, repeat yourself, or lose track of the time. So unless you are sure that none of those problems will apply, you should at least have a general outline of your talk, slide by slide.

Humor works well in nearly all settings, but bad taste does not. The only person you can make fun of is yourself, and that should only be done in very small doses.

PRACTICING YOUR TALK

Always practice your talk, preferably several times, in front of a sympathetic group of colleagues. For these practice sessions, you should use mock versions of your slides. The first session should be mainly for content. Did you include everything that needs to be presented? Is the general order of the presentation clear? What can be eliminated? Ask someone to time the talk.

After fixing any initial problems, have a second practice session for form and fluidity. Are the slides clear? Does the talk bog down in spots? Is there a connection between each slide and the next? Ask for specific comments about the slides themselves.

Finally, make your final slides and practice with them. If you have multicolored figures, make sure that the colors can be distinguished. Proofread for errors, using the projected slides. Then fix them. Sloppy slides are a sign of a sloppy scientist. If you discover a typo or mistake in a slide during a practice talk, either fix it right away (in the middle of the practice session), or make a written note to do so. It is easy to forget. One effective technique is to print a copy of the slides (four or six to a page to save paper!), and ask someone in the practice audience to take notes on those printed sheets. If, however, you discover an error after it is too late to make any changes, tell the audience, unless the error is trivial (e.g., the slide says the mean age was 71.4 years, and it should have been 71.6 years).

If you have never done so before, practice using a laser pointer. Use it sparingly—imagine that you have to pay $100 each time you turn it on. Avoid making frantic circles and squiggles. Do not use the pointer on every slide or to emphasize text. It should only be used to draw the audience's attention to an essential feature that would otherwise be difficult to notice, such as a feature in an image or a particular numeric result.

DEALING WITH ANXIETY

Rehearse both your talk and the question-and-answer session that will follow. Have a formal rehearsal, standing at the front of a medium-sized to large room, with an audience, even if it is only five or six people, in semi-darkness. Ask someone to watch for nervous mannerisms, such as a tendency to speed up (and ask that person to tell you about them in private!).

Even if you do not normally get nervous speaking before an audience, do not assume that stage fright will not strike when you least expect it. So just before the talk itself, use the rest room. Check your appearance in a mirror. Have a handkerchief or tissue to dry your hands and brow, if necessary. Bring a glass of water with you to the podium. A dry mouth can strike suddenly, and there is nothing more difficult than speaking when your mouth feels like the Gobi Desert. If that happens to you, take a 5-second break from your talk for a nice, refreshing sip. You, and everyone in the audience, will feel much better. To help prevent dry mouth, avoid, if possible, taking antihistamines and sympathomimetic medications before your talk.

Sprinkle friends in the audience, a few on each side, about five rows from the front. Do not expect your colleagues to anticipate this need; they will not, and will usually wind up hiding in the back of the room. Be direct: "It would help me a lot if you would sit in about the fifth row, on the left side as you enter the room." As you begin your talk, focus on these friends. Look at them long enough to elicit a nod or smile. Encouragement means just that—providing courage. You may also find it helpful to have a colleague sitting next to you as you wait your turn to speak.

Many speakers find that a small dose of a β-blocker helps ease anxiety. If you are thinking of using a β-blocker, be sure to "pretest" the dose a few days before, just to make sure you do not suffer any significant side effects.

Most important of all, prepare for questions. This is the part that many new investigators are most nervous about and least prepared for. Your coinvestigators may be too close to the project, and to you, to provide tough practice questions, unless you specifically ask them to do so.

THE TALK ITSELF

Most meeting organizers will send you instructions about what to do if you have an oral presentation, such as where and when to turn in your slides. Make sure your slides are labeled with your name, not just "Talk for Internal Medicine Meeting," which will be the same title everyone else will be using. Check that the presentation actually works. Get a memory stick and carry an extra copy of your talk with you. E-mail a copy of the slides to yourself before you leave for the meeting, so you can recover them while traveling if necessary.

Arrive at the session early. If you have not already done so, hand your slides to the projectionist. Introduce yourself to the chair(s) of the session. If you and your colleagues do not know them, do a literature review before the meeting to learn their areas of interest. Make small talk with them, as they will likely be looking for something to do as the attendees file into the room. As a bonus, if the session moderators get to know you, they may even become protective toward you and protect you from a persistent questioner.

Sit in an aisle seat, close to the speaker's podium. Listen to the talks that precede yours, so that you can incorporate previous speakers' work into your own presentation. If someone covers the same background or methodology you were planning to discuss, figure out how to shorten your talk appropriately.

ANSWERING QUESTIONS

If you appear gentle and humble, the audience will be on your side. Hostile questions will seem inappropriate or even nasty. So it is better to answer a question by saying, "I don't know," than to answer incorrectly. Practice ending your responses by making it clear that you have nothing more to say ("I hope that answers your question."), and asking for the next question ("Next question, please.").

While you may be asked some pretty strange questions, here are five basic ones that you can practice answering:

1. **Q:** Why didn't you do the study that I would have done?

   A: This one is easy to answer. Smile, and say something like, "That's an interesting idea, but not what we set out to do in this study."

2. Q: Why didn't you mention my previous work?

>   **A:** If you are familiar with the work, and it is good: "Thanks for pointing that out. I did not have time to discuss all the excellent studies on this question."

>   **A:** If you are familiar with the work, and it is not good: "Thanks for pointing that out. I did not have time to discuss all the previous studies on this question."

>   **A:** If you are not familiar with the work: "Thanks for pointing that out. I am not familiar with that study, but I will be sure to look into it."

3. Q: Could there be confounding (laboratory error, etc.)?

>   **A:** If you dealt with the concern: "That is an important concern, which we tried to minimize by doing…."

>   **A:** If you considered and rejected the concern: "We considered that possibility, but decided that it was unlikely because…."

>   **A:** If you did not consider the concern: "That is an interesting suggestion that we had not considered."

4. Q: Why didn't you use the "X" statistic (or the "Y" technique)? (This question has several variants, such as "Why didn't you measure quality of life using the instrument I just developed?")

>   **A:** If you did use it: "We did, and the results were very similar," or "We did, and the results changed slightly, and …," or "We did, and the results were different."

>   **A:** If you did not use it: "That is an interesting suggestion."

5. Q: Can your results be generalized?

>   **A:** "The most conservative interpretation is that our results apply only to two-humped camels. We are comfortable extrapolating to one-humped camels and llamas, but would be cautious about generalizing to all mammals."

Several other common types of problems may come up during the question-and-answer session. For instance, how do you respond when you do not know the answer? "That is an interesting question that I cannot answer." Because this reply goes against the natural tendency to answer even when one does not know, practice it a few times.

How do you respond when the questioner missed the answer during the presentation? "Perhaps I was not clear when I presented…."

What if you cannot understand the question, especially if the questioner is not fluent in English? "I am afraid I am having difficulty with your question. Perhaps we could discuss it after the session."

How do you respond when the questioner persists or is hostile? "Maybe we could continue this discussion after the session. Next question." Turn to the session chair for help. Part of that person's responsibility is to ensure that the question-and-answer session does not bog down. In this regard, it helps if the chair knows you, even if he or she just met you a few minutes before the session. If the chair does not step in, then turn and ask, "Who has the next question?"

What do you do when someone asks a two-part (or more) question? These are rude. (Sorry, but they are. Do not ask them of your colleagues; ask one question at a time. If you must ask two questions, say, "I have two questions. The first question is ..." and wait for the reply before asking a second.) It is very difficult to keep track of two questions. Fortunately, everyone in the audience knows this, and most will not remember both questions either. So do not worry about it. Answer one of the questions. Then, if you cannot remember the other one, say "Could you repeat the other question?" There is a good chance the questioner will have forgotten as well.

ADVICE FOR NON-ENGLISH SPEAKERS

Even investigators who read English well, and can write well enough to make their point, often have difficulty with spoken English. The combination of the extra anxiety of being in front of a room of strangers, plus concerns about having an accent, make public speaking a special challenge.

It is essential to be well prepared. Write out your talk in advance, and have a native English speaker (not just someone you think speaks well) review the talk and correct any errors in grammar or meaning. Then practice reading the corrected talk aloud, several times. Start when you are alone, then before a group of people. Ask them to stop you whenever they cannot understand what you are saying. Practice until you can make yourself understood. Sometimes you may need to rewrite sentences that contain words or phrases that are difficult for you to pronounce.

It will be easier to give your talk, which you can practice many times, than it will be to answer the subsequent questions. Especially if you are well rehearsed, the audience may overestimate your facility with English. They may assume that you are fluent, which may be far from the truth. If this applies to you, end your talk by saying: "Thank you for your attention. I will be happy to try to answer your questions, but English is not my first language. Please speak slowly and simply." Most people will be very sympathetic. If someone rushes through a difficult three-part question, no one in the audience will expect you to be able to answer.

If you have difficulty understanding a question, say "I am sorry, but I do not understand your question. Perhaps we can discuss it after the session."

SOME FINAL THOUGHTS

Many young investigators have a love–hate relationship with oral presentations. When they submit an abstract to a meeting, they fervently hope to be selected for an oral presentation. The first few days after submission are spent anticipating that the abstract will have a successful reception and envisioning the talk. This brief cheer may be followed by pessimism, as the shortcomings of the work become more apparent. Then if the abstract is chosen, a brief celebration ensues. Next comes completion of the analyses, which is often accompanied by the discovery that things are not quite the same as when the abstract was submitted. Planning the talk, making the slides, and even deciding what to wear are often fun; discovering an error on a critical slide at the last minute is not.

By the time of the talk, you may find yourself wondering whether it will turn out to be worth the intellectual and emotional effort you have expended. Will your hard work go for naught if you trip over a phrase or cannot answer a question clearly? What if there is no one in the audience? Why not just submit the manuscript?

Even if only 20 or 30 people hear your talk or see your poster, presenting your work in a public scientific forum is an important part of the process of becoming a full-fledged member of the community of clinical investigators. Like any rite of passage, the experience will be more valuable if you take the time to acknowledge your accomplishments and to appreciate the colleagues and mentors who have helped you.

CHECKLIST FOR

ORAL PRESENTATIONS

1. Does your presentation include all of the following slides: title and investigators, background, research question, methods, results, limitations, and conclusions?

2. Will all the information on all your slides be visible from the back of a darkened room?

3. Do you have no more than one slide for each minute of your talk?

4. Have you practiced and timed your talk?

5. Have you practiced answering difficult questions?

13

Choosing a Journal and Responding to Reviews

Most authors want their manuscript to be published in a most prestigious journal possible. They also hope that their work will be accepted and published expeditiously. On rare occasions, both these desires are fulfilled. More commonly, however, the more prestigious the journal to which you initially submit your manuscript, the longer the time before it is eventually accepted somewhere.

There are two reasons for the delay. First, prestigious journals are highly selective. Therefore, your manuscript is more likely to be rejected by such a journal—which may publish only 1 in 10 or 20 submissions—and the process of informing you may take several weeks or months. Second, even if a prestigious journal is interested in your work, the editors may require several versions before the manuscript meets their standards.

If you want to take a shot at a high impact, prestigious journal, then do so. But do not persevere in the face of repeated rejections. Accept the reality that if top-notch journals A and B were not interested in your work, it is unlikely that top-notch journal C will react differently.

CHOOSING A JOURNAL

Some investigators have a target journal in mind from the time they begin writing a manuscript and can prepare it accordingly. You will need a good deal of experience, however, before you develop a reliable sense of whether a journal is likely to accept your submission. The main advantage of targeting a manuscript is that different journals have slightly different rules about manuscript form and style. This is less of an issue now that most journals follow the "Uniform Requirements for Manuscripts Submitted to Biomedical Journals" (see Appendix A).

A more useful approach for new investigators is to write the best possible manuscript and then solicit advice about journals that might be appropriate. Begin by asking senior colleagues who regularly publish their research to read your manuscript and recommend three groups of journals: (1) Those that are likely to accept the manuscript (say, with a 60% likelihood or better); (2) those that offer a realistic possibility (say, 10% to 60%); and (3) others that seem unlikely but possible (>0% but

<10%). Ask them not to mention those that seem impossible. If you are in a hurry, submit the manuscript to one of the "likely to accept" journals. Otherwise, submit to one of the realistic possibilities.

Only rarely should you submit a manuscript to a journal in the long-shot (0% to 10%) category. Why? Unless you have brutally honest colleagues, you are unlikely to be told the truth about the quality of your manuscript. A manuscript that a colleague tells you is a long shot with a particular journal is not likely to be accepted, and the time and disappointment are usually not worth it.

If you do not have access to advice, then look at the 5 or 10 key references in your citations. What journal were they published in? Is your manuscript of comparable, lesser, or greater importance and quality? If you are not sufficiently familiar with the field to rate journals, then ask for help from your medical librarian, who can provide you with information about journal circulation and frequency of citation, both of which are rough indices of journal quality.

If you submitted the abstract from your study, consider the response it received. The manuscript from an abstract that was chosen as a plenary session at a major national meeting has more going for it than the manuscript describing the results of a study that was presented as a poster at a regional conference.

Finally, consider submitting your manuscript to a journal that you read regularly. This ensures that you know what kind of manuscripts and subject matter the journal publishes. The problem, of course, is that many authors read only one or two high-prestige journals. If you hope to be a serious investigator, you must develop the habit of being a regular reader of the most important journals in your research area.

Whether or not you are familiar with a journal, read the instructions to authors. If the journal does not accept review articles, or restricts articles to 3,000 words or less, do not submit a 30-page literature review or a 5,000-word masterpiece.

◆ WHAT TO PUT IN THE COVER LETTER

The basic format of the cover letter is simple.

> We are pleased to submit the enclosed manuscript, "Why we think you should publish our study," as a(n) (original article, review, letter to the editor, and so on) for publication in the *Journal of Friendly Editors and Reviewers*. This manuscript is entirely original, and it is not under review elsewhere. There is no overlap with other manuscripts that are in review. All authors take responsibility for the contents of the manuscript, including review and approval of this version, and satisfy the requirements for authorship. There are no relevant financial conflicts of interest. The corresponding author can be reached at
>
> First (or Last) Author, MD
>
> Mailing address
>
> Phone number
>
> Fax number
>
> E-mail address

What if the manuscript is not entirely original? You must explain how it differs from any previous version. Be aware that few editors will be interested in a manuscript that was originally addressed to a different audience ("The previous manuscript appeared in a pediatrics journal, not a radiology journal.") or that represents the same results with a slightly different twist ("Previous manuscripts have presented the 1-, 2-, and 3-year follow-up results; in this manuscript, we present the 4-year follow-up."). Similarly, if there might be overlap with another submitted manuscript (or one that is *in press* or recently published), be sure to discuss how the submitted manuscript represents a discrete body of work, and enclose copies of the potentially overlapping manuscript or manuscripts.

Financial conflicts are another issue that must be addressed. Most journals will require that you disclose relationships that you or any of the authors have with companies that may benefit from the publication of the manuscript.

Editors vary as to how much attention they pay to a cover letter that explains why you chose to submit your manuscript to their journal. It cannot hurt to explain your reasons, if you have good ones.

> Although this may appear to be a rather specialized topic, we make the point in the discussion that the results in this group of patients with a very rare inherited immunodeficiency syndrome are almost certainly applicable to patients with acquired defects in their immune systems.

> There have been six previous studies of this question (references 2 to 7 in the manuscript). However, all these studies failed to adjust for important confounders, such as smoking and use of alcohol, and so reached different conclusions from ours.

Always provide the name, address, phone number, fax number, and e-mail address for the corresponding author. If that person is going to be away for more than a few weeks, then provide an alternate. Make sure that the mailing address you provide is accessible to express mail services. Federal Express and the United Parcel Service, for instance, will not ship to post office boxes.

Finally, make sure that the letter or other submitted documentation addresses any other specific requirements that are unique to the journal. Some journals have what seems like an unending supply of forms to fill out and signatures to obtain before they will consider your manuscript. Do not ignore the forms in the hope that they can be filled out later. The editorial staff who receives your manuscript may not pass it on to the editors until all the paperwork is complete.

SUGGESTING REVIEWERS

It is always permissible to ask that a particular person review, or not review, your manuscript. Be aware, however, that the request may be ignored. If you know reviewers who are likely to be particularly hostile, ask that they not be sent the manuscript to review. This way, if the editor sends them the manuscript anyway, their comments will usually be discounted (not ignored, just discounted). But remember—if you had not mentioned their names, the editor may not have thought to send them the manuscript, and they may identify (or worse, say they have identified) a fundamental flaw in your manuscript, which the editor will be unable to ignore.

Always explain why you make a request, especially when there is someone whom you do not want to review your manuscript. There are a few acceptable reasons for someone to be excluded from the review process, including the need to protect confidential information, academic disputes, and previous personal problems.

Both our research groups have been working on this question for some time, and it has been our experience with the *Journal of Crummy Reviewers* that Drs. Slow and Poke have held on to manuscripts for several months while they redid the studies themselves.

We suggest in the manuscript that Dr. Lao-Ze's work is misleading and that her methodology is inadequate.

One of the authors previously worked in Dr. Harris Ment's laboratory and came close to filing a lawsuit against him.

Requesting particular reviewers is simple.

Drs. Baird and Crane are noted experts in the area and have recently published on the topic in (your journal, another prestigious journal).

THE MANUSCRIPT ITSELF

Your best chances for acceptance come with the editors' and reviewers' first impressions. The more your manuscript looks and reads like other articles in that journal, the better. Spend time "acquiring" a journal's style. If a journal rarely has articles with more than 2 or 3 tables, do not include 8 or 10 in your manuscript. If the journal has a particular way of presenting P values or spelling out abbreviations, use that form. Most of the time, these style points are in the "Instructions for Authors." Follow them as closely as possible.

Do not crowd your manuscript by extending the margins, or narrowing the space between lines, to keep the manuscript under the stipulated maximum length. A dense manuscript (see Chapter 14) is annoying to review and edit. Double-space all materials.

If you are sending "hard copy" of your manuscript (rather than an electronic version), send in the requested number of copies. Number the pages, the tables, and the figures. Put your name on everything.

The rush to publish often leads to mistakes. If you are a new investigator, a reviewer will regard a sloppy manuscript as evidence of sloppy work. Read your article before you send it in. Look at a printed copy, not just the computer screen. Do not trust a spell-checking program to find all the typographic errors. Have a friend, colleague, or relative read the article aloud, while you listen along with another copy. Look carefully for typographic errors and sentences that do not make sense. Check that the numbers in the tables are internally consistent. (Do they add up to the listed sum?) Compare the numbers in the abstract, text, and tables. Check that the references match the citations.

THE RESPONSE TO YOUR MANUSCRIPT

There are several basic types of responses to your manuscript. It may be accepted as it was submitted ("as is") or if you make a few minor corrections. You may be offered the chance to submit a revised version of the manuscript that addresses the reviewers' and editors' concerns about the previous version. The latter category includes those manuscripts that the journal thinks it is likely to accept if the authors make the requested changes and those that require more extensive revision and reevaluation, often by the original reviewers as well as the editors. Finally, a manuscript may be rejected with no opportunity offered to submit a revised version. This decision, which is discussed in more detail later in this chapter under the heading, "Dealing with Rejection," is final. The language will look like this:

> We are sorry that we cannot use your manuscript in the *Journal of Fussy Editors.*

> We regret to inform you that we are rejecting your manuscript for publication in the *Annals of Critical Reviewers.*

If your manuscript was accepted as submitted, or with only a few minor changes, rejoice. This often means that you did not aim high enough in choosing a journal! The editor's letter will include language like this.

> We are pleased to accept your manuscript for publication in the *International Journal of Medicine and Psychiatry.*

> If you will make the following changes, we will be pleased to accept your manuscript in the *Archives of Health Care Management.*

Only if you receive a letter officially accepting your manuscript can you list it as "in press" on your CV. At any point prior to that—even if you have received overwhelmingly favorable reviews and a glowing letter from the editor—the journal editors may still change their minds. Unless there is evidence of fraud, almost all journal editors will honor their commitment to publish an officially accepted manuscript, even if it is scooped between the time of acceptance and the time of publication.

The category of "revise and resubmit" is a bit grayer. Some journals do not distinguish between manuscripts that are likely to be accepted and those that truly need reevaluation (or if they do so, they keep the distinction to themselves). If the editors thought your manuscript was likely to be acceptable if some changes were made, they *may* tell you so with language like this:

> We are interested in your manuscript, and suggest the following changes in response to the concerns of our reviewers....

Another clue is that the editors may ask for a release of copyright, or give you a certain date by which they want the changes (so that they can use the manuscript in a particular issue). However, even with these sorts of comments, the editors usually do not guarantee publication, even if you make all the requested changes.

The next category involves an offer to submit a revised manuscript, with the clear expectation that the manuscript will be reviewed again. Usually, this category is reserved for those manuscripts that may not be acceptable even if all the suggested changes are made and all the reviewers' and editors' questions are answered. You may receive a letter with wording like this:

> Although your manuscript has merit, the reviewers and editors had several concerns that must be addressed before a decision can be made.

> We think that your manuscript may be of interest to our readers but request that you submit a revised version before we make a final decision.

> There are several concerns with the submitted manuscript, as pointed out in the comments from the reviewers and editors. Until we see your response, we cannot make a judgment about your manuscript.

If you cannot tell which category your manuscript is in, it may be worth calling the editorial office to find out.

RESPONDING TO COMMENTS

Read all the comments carefully, especially those from the editor because he or she is the ultimate decision maker, and failing to heed his or her suggestions is inadvisable. Number the comments and assess each one. Get to work on those that require new data or analyses. Do not assume that an explanation of why you did not change the manuscript will be sufficient. The editor or reviewer may decide that you ignored the recommendation. This usually results in a rejection, even if the initial reviews seemed positive.

Respond thoroughly to all comments. It is rarely appropriate to refuse suggestions from the editors. Although they may not be as expert as you are in the field, they know what they want in their journal. Therefore, if they think that the article is 50% too long, Figure 3 is not needed, and the discussion is confusing, make the recommended changes.

Indicate where and how the manuscript was changed. Include a cover letter numbering and detailing the editors' and reviewers' comments, your response to them, and any changes you made in the manuscript. Some journals request an "edited copy" with the deletions crossed out and the additions highlighted.

If you are an investigator who is junior enough to be reading this book, it is unlikely that you are in a position to argue with a reviewer. Calling him or her an ignoramus is unlikely to improve the reviewer's impression of your revised manuscript. Nor is it likely to win favor with the editor, who presumably chose the reviewer for his or her expertise. Resist the temptation to provide glib answers to what appear to be trivial comments. Take a deep breath, and respond politely.

> We considered the reviewer's suggestion that we redo the way we measured bone density in the cohort. The reviewer raised the important point as to whether we used the best available method to measure bone density. In response, we can only reply that at the time we started the study, the recommended technology was (unavailable, too expensive, too dangerous, of uncertain reliability, etc.).

> We had considered that possibility at the time we did the study, and based on a review of the literature (see references 21 and 22 in the manuscript) and a discussion with experts (Drs. Smart and Clever), we decided to use the methods in our study. In hindsight, we should have used the recommended methods; this is now acknowledged as a limitation of our study on page 15 in the revised version.

If you do not change the manuscript, say so and why. Provide cogent explanations. If a suggestion was not feasible, explain why.

> Because these data were not collected and the subjects are now dead, we are unable to ascertain previous history of birth trauma. We recognize that this is a limitation of our study and have added a discussion of this point (p. 23).

> We carefully considered the suggestion to delete Table 2, but believe that the information in that table is essential and cannot be covered in the text.

Sometimes, it is wise to offer to change the manuscript, even if you have not actually done so.

> Although we have not added these results to the manuscript—in the interest of saving space—we would be happy to do so should you wish. We could add a paragraph in the results and an additional figure, and expand our discussion of this topic.

OTHER CHANGES IN A REVISED MANUSCRIPT

Update the manuscript, if necessary, and correct mistakes from one version to the next. Always point such changes out.

> In re-reading, we noticed…. While these changes do not substantially affect….

> In checking our analyses, we found…. These differences have changed … and we have rewritten….

Failure to point out changes may have adverse consequences. A reviewer who notices changes that the authors did not acknowledge may write a hostile second review, including confidential comments to the editor. The reviewer may remember your name and judge you harshly in the future (and in many fields, there are a limited number of potential reviewers, so you may get the same one many times). A reputation for cutting corners may last your entire professional career.

Update the reference list if important new studies have been published. Tell the editor why you think your results still matter. A reviewer may think otherwise, but this at least gives you first crack at the editor.

Finally, treat the revised manuscript the same as a new submission. Check all the numbers. Look for typographic errors. Check the references.

EDITORIAL CHANGES

After an article is accepted, it must still be edited. Sometimes, this consists of correcting typographic and spelling errors, clarifying sentences, and changing the title of a figure or table. At other times, the editors may make much more extensive changes. If you disagree with the changes, you will have the opportunity to restore the original when you review the galleys or page proofs. But the editor and the publisher make the final decision.

DEALING WITH REJECTION

Rejection is tough, whether your manuscript is returned without review or is turned down after an extensive review process. The period that elapses between submission and the editor's response may give rise to false hopes. Encouragement by mentors and colleagues may do the same. Everyone knows someone who struck pay dirt the first time.

After opening the envelope containing a rejection letter, it is hard not to feel personally rebuffed and want to give up. You just spent several months working on your project, and it is understandable that you think your manuscript is terrific. Not everyone is going to agree with you, however, and it is rarely worth arguing with an editor about the decision—or asking your mentor to do so.

The harshest response is when a journal does not even send your manuscript for external review before rejecting it. Look on the bright side—at least you found out quickly and can move on to another journal. Until you gain more experience and acquire a better sense of what various journals are looking for—so that you can target your manuscripts more effectively—this is likely to happen often.

There are many reasons why a journal may have turned you down, including the design of the study, its execution, the statistical analyses, the presentation of the data, the importance of the research topic, the relevance of the results, the number of other manuscripts that the journal received that month, the perceived needs of the journal's readers, the editors' desire to balance the types of articles they publish, and, of course, the complete inability of the editors to recognize your masterpiece.

So relax. Use the criticism in the reviews to improve the manuscript. Suppose you received a firm rejection letter with no reviews and no indication of the manuscript's problems. This tells you that the editors would not have been interested in your manuscript even if the reviewers had liked it. Almost any of the reasons in the previous paragraph may apply. If you want to narrow the list, send a brief note to the editors with the manuscript number, asking politely for an explanation (not challenging the decision). If you have a specific question, ask.

> You recently turned down my manuscript (No. 1,234) without comment. As I am interested in submitting the manuscript to another journal, would you be willing to let me know, in a few words or sentences, the main problems with the manuscript? Was it because the manuscript was too long?/the study was not a randomized trial?/too many subjects dropped out?

However, it is not the editors' job to provide you with detailed feedback about your manuscript. Everything you get other than a simple yes or no is gravy.

Journal editors do not count reviewers' votes and decide based on majority rule. Reviewers serve in an advisory capacity to the editors. Journals are not obligated to accept an article even if two or three reviews are favorable. They do not have to obtain additional reviews if you do not like the ones they obtained, and they do not need to provide you with a detailed description of the thought process behind their decision. Moreover, reviewers usually provide a separate set of confidential comments to the editors. Therefore, although the comments for the authors may have appeared neutral or even favorable, those for the editors may have read something like this:

> Fine as far as it goes, but not of any interest to the field.

> Methodologically sound, clinically meaningless.

> So poorly done that I did not bother making detailed comments for the authors.

> Authors are naïve about research; I did not know where to begin in making specific suggestions.

> Superb methods; should be published in another journal, however.

> Not as well done as the article by Schweitzer et al. on the same topic that just appeared in the *Journal of Neurology.*

Sometimes, the reviewers working in a particular field think a manuscript is terrific, but neither the manuscript nor the reviews convince the editors that the manuscript will be of interest to the journal's readers.

Suppose you submitted your manuscript to a top-notch journal and received a few favorable reviews, but the editors rejected the manuscript anyway. The rejection letter mentions editorial priorities or indicates that the journal receives far more manuscripts than it can possibly accept. Should you complain? What if you received two reviews, one favorable and the other not favorable? Should you request another review? What if the journal took 6 months to reject your manuscript? Should you demand that it be published because of the unconscionable delay? Should you pester the editorial staff for additional information? Probably not. Your time will be better spent preparing the manuscript for submission to another journal.

Most journals do not have a formal appeals process for rejected manuscripts because it would rarely be worth the trouble. Few rejected manuscripts are close calls. Those that are were usually considered in some detail before a decision was made. Only if you have some important new information that might change the editorial decision is an appeal warranted, and then only in the form of a brief note:

> You recently turned down my manuscript (No. 2,345) for publication in your journal. Since the time I submitted the manuscript there have been several important developments in the field. First, we have studied another 54 patients, with similar results, which are now both clinically and statistically significant. Second, Redo and Undo have retracted their article in *Hypothesis and Theory,* whose findings were cited by the reviewer as the key reason why our manuscript was not important. Because of these developments, would you be willing to reconsider a revised manuscript?

Politeness is essential. Journal editors are aware that they are fallible, but prefer to be reminded of it in a quiet voice.

If you do decide to protest a decision, make sure you are clear about your goals. If all you want to do is ventilate your frustrations, and are planning to send the manuscript elsewhere, then open your window and scream. If you genuinely want the manuscript to appear in that journal, then write a gentle note saying something like this:

> I was very disappointed to receive your letter of April 1 rejecting my manuscript (No. 11-628). I had hoped that the *New Brunswick Journal* would publish it, and I wonder if there is anything I can do to persuade you to reconsider that decision.

Then provide a few specific reasons why you think the manuscript is worthwhile. You may want to include a *brief* response to the gist of the reviewers' or editors' comments:

> The main concern of the reviewers was that the study was not double-blinded. Actually, it was; we neglected to mention this in the methods.

> The reviewers seemed to be concerned with the methods we used to measure parathyroid hormone. Since the time we submitted the study, we have performed analyses comparing our methods with the standard radioimmunoassay and have found an intraclass correlation of 0.95.

> The editors indicated that the manuscript did not meet the priority of the journal, given that there have been several previous studies in this area. We would like to emphasize that we studied more patients than all the previous studies combined, and our results run counter to the prevailing dogma.

The chances are not great (actually, they are quite small) that the editors will change their minds, but at least you will have provided them a graceful way of doing so.

The worst option is to call the office and berate whoever answers the phone while you demand to speak with the editors. This will accomplish little except to give you a reputation for being difficult. Even if the editor does call you back, the manuscript's file is likely to contain a note from the staff that says, "Warning: difficult author."

SUBMITTING TO ANOTHER JOURNAL

After a rejection, it is best to get back on the horse. Do not allow yourself to wallow in self-pity while your manuscript gathers dust. Get to work on a revised version that day. The longer you wait, the harder it will be to get going. At some point, even the most compelling reasons (such as a pending promotion or grant) will not suffice.

If the manuscript was reviewed and then rejected, approach it as if you had received a "revise and resubmit" letter. Go back in this chapter to the sections titled "Responding to Comments" and "Other Changes in a Revised Manuscript", and follow the directions for manuscript revision. Select a new target journal, confirm that your manuscript fits its editorial needs, and restyle it so that it looks like it belongs in the new journal.

Do not just make some new copies of the manuscript and send it to another journal. You may get the same reviewers, and having failed to follow their past suggestions will not help your cause.

What about including previous reviews of the manuscript when you submit to another, presumably less prestigious, journal? So long as your new manuscript addresses the previous reviewers' concerns (and you tell the new editors how), there is nothing to lose by doing this. However, if the previous set of reviewers identified what they thought was a major problem with the study, then you are taking a risk unless you address—and, preferably, fix—the problem. At best, the editors may decide to rely on the previous reviews to save time. At worst, the editors will ignore the other reviews, and you are back where you would have been anyway. All that can happen is that the editor will be insulted at receiving a hand-me-down. But most editors have better things to do than worry about the underlying meaning of your decision to send them a manuscript that was rejected by journal X.

✓ CHECKLIST FOR

MANUSCRIPT SUBMISSION

1. Does the cover letter include the important details about how to contact the authors?

2. Do you provide reasons if you suggest certain reviewers or ask that certain reviewers be excluded?

3. Does the manuscript look like it belongs in the journal? Did you follow the rules for submission??

Responding to Editors

1. Did you include a cover letter that listed all the comments and your responses to them? Did you mention where your responses appear in the revised manuscript?

2. Did you mention any other changes in the manuscript?

3. Are your responses polite, almost to the point of obsequiousness?

4. Did you re-read the manuscript, just as if it were a new submission?

14 Suggestions for Writing Well

Writing, even writing poorly, does not come easily to most investigators. Some lack the activation energy to get started. Others have a half dozen manuscripts in various stages of completion that they never manage to finish. Whatever the problem, you can improve your productivity and your writing.

First, decide whether it is worth your time and effort to write the manuscript. If you are having a hard time motivating yourself to start, perhaps it is because you do not have much to say. Does the world really need the manuscript? If not, cut your losses and move on to another project.

Next, make sure you are familiar with the software program that you will need to produce your manuscript. Learn how to make tables (either in a word-processing program or in a spreadsheet) and figures (either in a spreadsheet or in presentation software). Take advantage of any spell-checking capabilities; make sure you spell medical words correctly when you add them to the dictionary. Use a bibliography program that will automatically number and format your references. Learn how to download references electronically into the program so that you do not have to key them in manually.

Finally, you cannot write well if you do not write at all. Do not fuss over the first draft of a manuscript. Just write, without worrying about style, brevity, spelling, grammar, or clarity. Prepare a draft that includes a title page, each section of the manuscript, and mock tables and figures. Add your name, a running title, the page number, and the date at the top of each page. Start each section on a new page. The more the draft looks like a manuscript, the prouder you will feel, and the more likely it will be that you and your coauthors will be willing to invest additional time in improving it. This works even if some of the sections consist of nothing more than the word *pending*.

Furthermore, you cannot write well if you do not *read* what you have written. Print a copy of the first draft. Read it to make sure that you have not left anything out. Make the necessary additions to the next draft, incorporate them into the word-processed version, and print the revised manuscript. Each version will be better than its predecessor, and the incremental improvements will encourage you to proceed.

When you think you have a nearly complete draft containing all the scientific material, print another copy and sharpen a pencil. Cross out every paragraph that is not necessary. Delete every extra sentence within the remaining paragraphs, and finally, the extraneous words within the remaining sentences. Underline everything that is not crystal clear, and write "Huh?" in the margin. Circle words that do not make sense. Put an arrow before every paragraph that does not flow logically from its predecessor and write "Segue?" Sharpen another pencil, and begin clarifying the ambiguities, replacing the awkward words and phrases, and filling in the missing links.

Style will be the objective for the next two or three drafts of the manuscript. But if you never learned how to write well, or are someone for whom English is a second language, do not fuss over this aspect. Hire a copy editor to do it for you.

When you think you are through, print another version and read it carefully for typographical and spelling errors. Make sure that the numbers make sense. Are they consistent between the methods and results? Between the text and tables? Between the results and discussion?

ADVICE FOR AUTHORS FOR WHOM ENGLISH IS A SECOND LANGUAGE

If you are a non–English-speaking author, do not submit a manuscript to an English-language journal until it has been read and edited by a native English speaker who understands the scientific content. Do not assume that just because someone speaks and writes English better than you do that they are fluent in the language. Furthermore, do not assume that someone who is fluent in English knows enough about the science in your manuscript to be able to help you. You need to find someone who is both *fluent* and *qualified scientifically* so that they can help you state your ideas, methods, findings, and conclusions clearly. Remember that journal editors do not enjoy reviewing manuscripts that are difficult to understand, and reviewers do not like having to read them because they take more time. Therefore, manuscripts describing good or even excellent work may not even be reviewed because the English is poor.

Where can you find someone to help you? That depends a bit on whether you are physically located in an English-speaking country. If you are, there should be no shortage of potential helpers. Often, there are students doing internships (or waiting to apply to medical school or graduate school) working as research assistants or technicians. Offer to cook them dinner or take them to lunch.

If you are not in an English-speaking country, you may have to look a bit longer to find someone who fits the bill. Best of all would be someone you worked with while training, especially if you spent some time doing so in an English-speaking country. Next, ask colleagues who have been successful at getting an article published in prestigious journals whether they know anyone appropriate. Another possibility is someone who is on sabbatical at your institution or someone you met at a scientific meeting. Be prepared to offer something valuable—like tickets to a concert or a medical textbook—in return. Finally, there are many professional medical writers and editors whose services are available for reasonable fees. (Unless you are famous, writing is a poorly remunerated occupation.)

If you do get help writing your manuscript, please do not automatically make your helper a coauthor on the manuscript. If all they did was help you prepare a grammatically correct version of the manuscript, they have not earned authorship rights (see Chapter 10).

AIMING FOR CLARITY

What seems clear to you may be impenetrable to others. There are a few basic principles to follow to ensure the clarity of your manuscript.

Know the Audience

Make sure you write your manuscript at a level appropriate for readers of your target journal. This principle is especially applicable to the introduction. Do not assume that because you know something, the reviewers, editors, and readers will also know it. If your work is at or near the cutting edge, other investigators and clinicians—even those in the same field—may not be as familiar with the area as you are.

If you are not sure that your paper will connect with your audience, pick up a few recent issues of the journal you hope will accept your manuscript. Read articles in areas about which you know little. How much background knowledge did they assume? How much did they spell out for the reader? The answers to these two questions will provide you with a baseline against which you can compare your manuscript.

Avoid Density

Dense pages—ones on which abbreviations, numbers, *P* values, and technical terms appear in profusion—are tough to read. No one *wants* to read them; no one *can* read them; no one *will* read them. Take a look at your manuscript. If there are sections of text that you cannot read aloud to a friend with a nontechnical background, change them.

It may be tempting to use abbreviations because they make your manuscript shorter. But you should only use abbreviations, such as EKG and DNA, that are in such common use they are as well or better known than the terms they represent. Do not assume that the world uses the same abbreviations and acronyms you do; they tend to be remarkably specific to single institutions or fields. You should almost never have a sentence with more than one abbreviation, so choose the most important one carefully. Better yet, leave them all out.

Change:

The effects of NSAIDs on PG synthesis in the GI tract are mediated through the COX system.

There were 17 patients with CHF, 11 with CHD, 23 with COPD, and 4 with CRF.

To:

The effects of nonsteroidal anti-inflammatory drugs on prostaglandin synthesis in the gastrointestinal tract are mediated through the cyclooxygenase (COX) system.

There were 17 patients with congestive heart failure, 11 with coronary heart disease, 23 with chronic obstructive lung disease, and 4 with chronic renal failure.

Although spelling out an abbreviation takes more space, it is usually easier to read the entire phrase than to translate mentally while reading.

Avoid pseudo-abbreviations such as "Groups 1, 2, and 3." Instead, develop code names, such as "Asthma, Bronchitis, and Emphysema" or "Cirrhosis without renal failure, Cirrhosis with renal failure, or Renal failure only."

The same guidelines hold true for paragraphs full of numbers. Your manuscript will be clearer if you put the numbers in tables and use the text to explain the tables, not to repeat them.

Eschew Vagueness When the Details Matter; Eschew Precision When They Do Not

Provide the appropriate level of detail. Avoid sentences that are too vague to be meaningful.

> ***Vagueness:***
>
> The treatment group did better than the control group ($P < 0.05$). Subgroup analyses found no differences.

Also avoid being overly precise.

> ***Excessive Precision:***
>
> When compared with the placebo group, the RR of gastrointestinal upset during the study in the group treated with controlazine 50 mg tablets was 0.518 (95% confidence interval 0.346 to 0.776).
>
> When the results were analyzed separately in men and in women, in those with recent abdominal surgery or not, and those with or without a history of peptic ulcer disease, the results were similar ($P = 0.36$, $P = 0.26$, and $P = 0.78$, respectively, using a test for the homogeneity of the odds ratio).

> ***Better:***
>
> When compared with the placebo group, only half as many patients (relative risk = 0.52; 95% confidence interval: 0.35 to 0.78) in the controlazine group had gastrointestinal upset.
>
> When analyzed separately in men and in women, in those with or without recent abdominal surgery, and in those with or without a history of peptic ulcer disease, the results were similar (all P for interaction >0.25).

Use Topic Sentences to Begin Each Paragraph

Let the reader know what to expect. Each section of the manuscript has its own type of topic sentence. The Introduction and Discussion sections are mainly about ideas, so introduce the key concepts.

> The reasons why coronary artery disease becomes more common in women after menopause are not certain.
>
> Most investigators rely on self-report to ascertain quality of life.

The paragraphs in a Methods section are usually introduced by the general area, such as subjects, measurements, and analysis, and then by subtopics.

> At a baseline exam, we asked subjects....
>
> We reviewed medical records....
>
> Using serum obtained at the initial examination, we measured....
>
> We ascertained the incidence of developmental problems by....

Topic sentences in the Results section are more factual.

> Of the 102 subjects, 18 were readmitted from nursing homes.
>
> During 3.2 years of follow-up, we identified 67 patients who developed....
>
> The main predictors of adverse outcomes were....
>
> When analyzed as a continuous variable....
>
> Adjusting for potential confounders had little effect.

Segue, Segue, Segue

Look for the connections between the ideas in your manuscript, and use words that link those ideas to join paragraphs together. Linking words and phrases include *however, indeed, rather, moreover, on the other hand, by contrast, in comparison, surprisingly,* and *consistent with.* Here are some segue phrases you can use to start sentences in the Discussion section.

> We found....
>
> We believe this means that....
>
> An alternative explanation is that....
>
> These results are consistent with....
>
> We also found....
>
> Our study has several strengths compared with....
>
> Our study has limitations also....
>
> Despite these limitations....
>
> In conclusion....

Keep Comparisons Together

Avoid separating the groups that are being compared. Do not interpose long phrases.

> ***Change:***
>
> There were more cases of esophageal cancer in our follow-up study of patients with Barrett's esophagus than there were cases of gastric cancer.
>
> ***To:***
>
> In our follow-up study of patients with Barrett's esophagus, there were more cases of esophageal cancer than gastric cancer.
>
> ***Even Better:***
>
> Patients with Barrett's esophagus were more likely to develop esophageal cancer than gastric cancer.

Because lists can be difficult to follow, you should avoid them. If that is impossible, then start the list with one-word phrases, then two-word phrases, then longer phrases, followed by compound phrases. If necessary, break the list into two sentences.

Awkward:

Hip fractures are more common in women than men, expensive, painful, and sometimes fatal.

Hip fractures often result in loss of independence or nursing home placement, may lead to chronic disability, and cause acute pain.

Easier to Follow:

Hip fractures are expensive, painful, and sometimes fatal. They are more common in women than in men.

Hip fractures cause acute pain, may lead to chronic disability, and often result in loss of independence or nursing home placement.

Whatever you do, keep the positives together and the negatives together.

Disorganized:

Subjects with myocardial infarction were less likely to be married, older, drank less alcohol, were better educated, and were more likely to smoke.

Clearer:

Subjects with myocardial infarction were older, better educated, and more likely to smoke and drink. They were less likely to be married or to drink alcohol.

Do not use different terms to express the same idea. Suppose you define *mildly ill* as having less than three symptoms, *moderately ill* as having three to six symptoms, and *severely ill* as having more than six symptoms. Stick with those terms. Do not switch among them.

Change:

Moderately ill patients were more likely to be hospitalized than those with fewer than three symptoms. Those with seven or more symptoms had an average time to recovery of 6.2 days.

To:

Moderately ill patients were more likely to be hospitalized than those with mild disease. Those who were severely ill had an average time to recovery of 6.2 days.

ACHIEVING BREVITY

Shorter is almost always better in a manuscript. A short manuscript is easier to write, easier to read, and easier to review. Although the basic techniques of achieving brevity have been discussed in the individual chapters, here are a few reminders. In the Results section, text, tables, and figures should be complementary. In the

Introduction and Discussion sections, synthesize the results of previous studies. Do not repeat methods in the results or results in the discussion.

Your best pruning tools are a sharp pencil and the delete command on your word processor. If you worry that as soon as you delete a paragraph, you will suddenly remember why you previously considered it critical, then paste the offending paragraph at the end of your text and leave it there until the final draft.

Eliminating sentences that are repeated in the abstract, introduction, results, and discussion is a quick way of shortening a manuscript. No one will miss the extra words. Do not let concerns that your manuscript may be too short inhibit your editing. Nor should you include filler material solely to lengthen a manuscript. Remember that no paper is too short.

DEVELOPING A STYLE

Scientific writing tends to be dry. Metaphors, similes, oxymorons, alliteration, and all the other literary devices whose names you no longer remember do not matter much. Although this may be lamentable, scientific writing can still have style. Unadorned, snappy, and crystal clear are the attributes of a well-written manuscript.

Verbs

Use the correct verb tense in each section of the manuscript. Use the *present tense* to describe the background in the introduction and to refer to the implications of your study in the discussion.

> Renal tubular acidosis often manifests as.... This study establishes the importance of.... One explanation for these differences is that....

Use the *past tense* to describe what you did in the Methods section and what you found in the results. In discussion, the past tense should be used when referring to previous studies or to your study's results, which you just presented.

> We randomly assigned.... We measured.... We analyzed....

> During the course of the study, 245 subjects had myocardial infarctions. Events were twice as frequent among those with high blood pressure.

> We found that.... By comparison, Kim et al. reported that....

The specific limitations and strengths of the study should also be presented in the past tense.

> We enrolled only subjects with a previous history of....

> Although we measured....

Generally, use the *active voice.* Active verbs say who did what to whom, rather than what was done to someone or something.

> ***Passive Voice:***
>
> The effect was estimated....

Active Voice:

We estimated the effect of ....

The passive voice also has a place. Use it for variety because reading the same sentence construction over and over gets dull.

Repetitive:

We enrolled .... We collected .... We measured sleep apnea by .... We analyzed ....

Varied:

We enrolled ... we measured .... Sleep apnea was measured by .... We analyzed ....

The passive voice also works when the action (not the subject) is being emphasized.

Patients who did not have phones were excluded.

The emphasis is on the process of exclusion, as opposed to who did the excluding or the details of who was excluded. By contrast, if stated as "we excluded patients without phones," the decision seems stern, almost mean-spirited.

Some authors have such pathologic fear of the passive voice that they use the verb "exist" as a substitute. This almost always results in a poorly written sentence.

Awkward:

There exist several previous studies of this question.

Replace by:

There are several previous studies of this question.

Do Not Stake Claims

Avoid bragging about having the first, the best, the biggest, or the most rigorous study. Not only can you rarely be sure but also why toot your horn? Leave these phrases for the reviewers and the editorialist. Let your work stand on its merits.

Bragging:

This phenomenon has never been previously reported in the English-language literature that we reviewed since 1980 using the keywords *angina* and *penicillin.*

Factual:

Treatment of angina with penicillin reduced symptoms in our subjects.

Avoid Using Confusing Words

Using *respectively* may seem to save words, but, like using abbreviations, it actually slows down the reader, who must check to see which number refers to which group.

Confusing:

The rates in the four groups (young men and women, older men and women) were 10%, 13%, 8%, and 21%, respectively.

Straightforward:

The rates were 10% in young men, 13% in young women, 8% in older men, and 21% in older women.

The phrase "we feel …" is not appropriate unless you are describing an emotion.

Probably Inappropriate:

We feel that this was the appropriate test to use.

Probably Appropriate:

We believe that this was the appropriate test to use.

Possibly Appropriate:

We feel badly that in these previous studies we forgot to measure body weight.

Demographic is an adjective, not a noun. Use *demographic characteristics* to refer to age, sex, and race or ethnicity, and *clinical characteristics* to refer to medical history and examination findings. Do not use terms such as *diabetics* and *asthmatics* to describe people with these medical conditions; use terms such as *diabetic patients* and *patients with asthma* instead. The word *database* should be used rarely because one rarely studies a database.

Do not anthropomorphize your study, as in "Our study found …." or "Our study showed …." The study did none of those things; you and the other investigators did.

Significant means *statistically significant.* If that is not your intent, use *substantial, large, important, notable, meaningful, valuable, or noteworthy.* Do not say "significant differences" unless you have also provided the direction and size of the difference, and an estimate of its precision. You need not provide the *P* value (or the confidence interval) in the discussion if you included it in the results.

Random means selected according to a prespecified rule in instances when the probability of selection is known. If that meaning does not apply, use *haphazard, nonsystematic,* or *convenience* to describe your sample.

An *average* is the mean of a group of numbers—the sum divided by the count. Do not use average to describe something else; use *typical, usual,* or *ordinary.*

Normal may mean "following a normal distribution" or "within a set of acceptable bounds." When these two possibilities can be confused, use *normally distributed* or *within normal limits,* as appropriate. Never use normal to mean typical or healthy.

Data are plural. Practice writing and saying this sentence: My data are better than your data; mine are better than yours. *Data* and *studies* are not synonyms. If there are few studies, say so; do not say that there are few data to support a particular position.

Do not say "over a 3-year period"; say "during a 3-year period." Comparisons are made *between* two groups but *among* three or more groups.

Which is often misused. Change which to *that* unless doing so clearly does not make sense. There are formal grammatical rules for deciding between which and that, but this technique usually works just as well.

Keep an eye open for unneeded fillers *(the fact that, in fact, in order to, with respect to, with regard to, regarding, the occurrence of, the nature of, it has been shown that),* and for phrases and big words where small words will do. Change *numerous* to *many, a number of* to *several, the vast majority* to *most, previous to this study* to *before,* and *every single* to *each.*

Trends and What They Are

The word *trend* has two common meanings in clinical research. One is to indicate a result that is oh-so-close to being statistically significant.

> There was a trend for cardiologists to order more PSA levels than internists did ($P = 0.08$).

This is flabby writing. Just state what you observed, with an emphasis on the effect size.

> Cardiologists ordered PSA levels in 52% of male patients; internists obtained levels 36% of the time ($P = 0.08$).

Another use of *trend is* to indicate a "dose–response" effect, usually by using a specific statistical test. This usage is acceptable.

> A χ^2 test for trend was significant: With increasing educational level, the risk of stroke declined.

> There was a significant trend between dose of narcotic analgesia (on a log scale) and pain relief.

The Abbreviations e.g. and i.e.

E.g. is the Latin abbreviation for *exempli gratia,* meaning "for example." The abbreviation *i.e.* stands for *id est,* which means "that is." These two abbreviations are not synonyms. Use *e.g.* when providing an example or two; the presumption is that there are other examples. Use *i.e.* to provide a more exact or complete definition of the prior phrase.

> There were several subjects with solid tumors (e.g., lung cancer, breast cancer).

> There were several subjects with solid tumors (i.e., lung cancer, breast cancer, colon cancer, or stomach cancer).

The second example implies that there were no other types of solid tumor included. Most journals use *e.g.* and *i.e.* within parenthetical phrases, sometime leaving out the periods but always including the comma. The full English phrase (for example, that is) should be used in nonparenthetical sentences:

> We did not include patients who did not speak English (i.e., those who could not understand the question, "Do you speak English well enough to shop in department stores?").

> Only those measurements that were clearly invalid, for example, those showing serum potassium levels below 1.8 mEq/L, were repeated.

Vague Adjectives and Adverbs

You would not write "a whole lot greater," so why write "*dramatically* greater?" unless referring to Shakespeare?

Higher and *lower* should be used sparingly, unless you are referring to temperature or other scales. Instead, use *more* and *less, greater* and *lesser, heavier* and *lighter*. This rule is often violated, however, as in "hemoglobin levels were higher in the cases than in the controls."

Be careful about *increased* and *decreased*. It is easy to misinterpret these two words as implying that something was measured more than once in the same subjects.

Misleading:

After 2 years of treatment, the mean glycosylated hemoglobin level was increased in diabetic patients treated with oral agents compared with those treated with insulin.

More Accurate:

After 2 years of treatment, the mean glycosylated hemoglobin level was greater in diabetic patients treated with oral agents than in those treated with insulin.

Avoid using *males* and *females*. Use more specific terms such as *men* and *women,* or *boys* and *girls,* or *male rabbits* and *female rabbits.* Also be wary of unintentionally funny phrases, such as "black and white men." Use "black men and white men." Beware of inadvertent juxtapositions of rodents and humans: "The effects of ketoconazole differed in male rats and in men."

WRITING NUMBERS AND FORMULAS

Most journals will not allow you to begin a sentence with an Arabic number.

Unacceptable:

116 subjects were enrolled. 23 patients died during the study.

Acceptable:

We enrolled 116 subjects. During 2 years of follow-up, 23 patients died.

Be consistent in how you present confidence intervals. Do not forget to indicate what sort of confidence interval you are presenting (e.g., 95%).

Acceptable for Confidence Intervals:

1.2 to 2.4   (1.2, 2.4)   (1.2–2.4)

The last version (1.2–2.4) uses an en dash (Ctrl minus sign). The en dash poses a problem if one or more of the intervals is a negative number; in that case, separate the intervals with a comma or the word *to*, and use a + sign to indicate that the sign has changed.

−10% to +5%   −10%, +5%

The same principle holds for means and standard deviations. Use the same format throughout. Usually, you will want to indicate in the methods that continuous data are presented as mean ± SD (or whichever format you choose).

Acceptable for Means and Standard Deviations:

45.3 ± 23.1   45.3 (23.1)   45.3 (*SD* 23.1)

Learn to use (Insert Symbol menu) the special characters ≥, ≤, and ±, rather than underlining >, <, or +. Add spaces before and after mathematical symbols. Change 6±1 to 6 ± 1 and change *P*=0.02 to *P* = 0.02. The additional spaces make the symbol easier to read. Use a "leading zero" before a decimal point (0.02, not .02), but leave out the zero after a decimal point unless relevant (e.g., 112, not 112.0); getting in the habit of doing so helps prevent medical errors.

Many journals require that numbers <10 be written out (e.g., four, not 4) unless decimal points are involved (e.g., 3.2).

OVERCOMING WRITER'S BLOCK

Almost all authors suffer occasionally from writer's block, the inability to put thoughts about a project into words. This malady is probably responsible for thousands of unwritten manuscripts. It is also the source of much distress among research teams, if the designated author's problems in making progress on a manuscript result in delays, but no one feels comfortable assigning the topic to another investigator on the team.

First, realize that you are in good company. The thought of sitting down before a blank notepad or an empty computer screen and creating a 3,000-word manuscript, with 4 tables, 3 figures, 40 references, and an abstract, intimidates many experienced authors.

Approach the problem systematically. Make a list of what needs to be accomplished, such as the sections of the manuscript, mock tables and figures, a list of key references, and the title page. Decide in what order you are going to do them. Sometimes the discussion and introduction are left for last because many investigators find them the hardest sections to write.

Assemble your materials in a single folder or pile. It will be much easier to write if you do not have to spend 20 minutes reassembling your materials each time. When you find an important reference, a key page in the operations manual, or essential printouts from the data analysis, label them clearly so you can remember why they are important when you look at them 6 weeks later.

Set aside 30 minutes every day, or every few days, as writing time. Preferably this will be early in the day, rather than late in the afternoon or evening when you are exhausted. Set a goal for each day, however modest ("Today, I will write the paragraph for the Methods section about how we enrolled the subjects."). Close the door to your office, and do not answer the phone or your pager.

Some authors prefer to set aside an entire day or two to write a manuscript. This technique works fine if you can do it, but most people who suffer from writer's block find it intimidating to imagine writing for an entire day. It can also be discouraging if you are unsuccessful; then you feel like you wasted a large block of time.

Write incrementally. Begin with the methods, then the results. For many investigators, these are the easiest parts of a manuscript to write because they are mostly science with little composition. Then add a paragraph of introduction and two paragraphs of discussion. Print a copy and casually jot down some notes on the printed version. Next, add these notes to the word-processed document. Print and admire. Add a few more notes. Repeat.

If even that is too hard, start with the design (a prospective study). Add the subjects (200 patients in the clinic), then the measurements ("We asked subjects about alcohol consumption and followed them for admission with pancreatitis."), then the analysis ("We estimated the risk of admission ..."). Write one paragraph at a time. The paragraph is the basic unit of your manuscript. If you are able to write one paragraph—and you can—then you will be able to write another. A paragraph takes a simple form. It covers one thought, rarely two, examined from a few angles. Begin with a topic sentence that explains what will follow.

Sometimes dictating your ideas into a tape recorder can help. If you have presented the study results already—for example, at a meeting or to your research group—you may find it simpler to say what you want to write than to write it. Then transcribe your dictation or have someone do it for you. While the spoken word rarely reads well, no matter how eloquent it sounded, at least you have a start.

Involve your coauthors at an early stage. As soon as you have something that looks even vaguely like a manuscript, send it around for comments. Give authors a specific assignment, such as "Mollie: Please describe the methods for the radioimmunoassay here. Stuart said you would know."

If none of those ideas helps, use one of the templates in this book. Even if they seem irrelevant to your subject matter, by changing the nouns and verbs you will have a start on the process.

There is another variety of writer's block—the inability to finish a manuscript. Among the many subtypes of this problem are endless tinkering with tables, never getting around to writing the conclusion, and being not quite able to find time to assemble the references. If your behavior can be described by any of these subtypes, then you will have to set deadlines, just as your teachers did for you in the past. If you tend to ignore your own deadlines, then have them set by your mentor or department chair.

Procrastination behaviors can often be attributed to a fear that the manuscript will be rejected. If you recognize that problem in yourself, remember that almost every manuscript will eventually find a better home than your file cabinet. The subjects in your study participated with the expectation that they were helping medical science. If nothing else convinces you to finish the manuscript, that should.

✔ CHECKLIST FOR

WRITING WELL

1. Is the manuscript (style, contents, and length) aimed appropriately at the intended audience? Does it look like the articles that have been published in the journal to which you are submitting it?

2. If English is your second (or third) language, has your manuscript been reviewed carefully by someone who is a native English speaker and is scientifically qualified to understand the content?

3. Have you deleted all extraneous material, unnecessary precision, and repetitive text?

4. Does each paragraph make sense on its own and fit well with its neighbors?

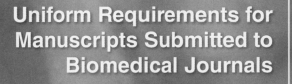

Uniform Requirements for Manuscripts Submitted to Biomedical Journals

An updated version of the complete text, including information on conflict of interest and the protection of human subjects, can be found at the Web site of the International Committee of Medical Journal Editors, www.ICMJE.org.

We have reproduced parts of the document—Manuscript Preparation and Manuscript Submission—modified slightly.

MANUSCRIPT PREPARATION

Editors and reviewers spend many hours reading manuscripts, and therefore appreciate receiving manuscripts that are easy to read and edit. Much of the information in a journal's Instructions to Authors is designed to accomplish that goal in ways that meet each journal's particular editorial needs. The following information provides guidance in preparing manuscripts for any journal.

General Principles

The text of observational and experimental articles is usually (but not necessarily) divided into the following sections: Introduction, Methods, Results, and Discussion. This so-called IMRAD structure is not an arbitrary publication format but rather a direct reflection of the process of scientific discovery. Long articles may need subheadings within some sections (especially Results and Discussion) to clarify their content. Other types of articles, such as case reports, reviews, and editorials, probably need to be formatted differently.

Electronic formats have created opportunities for adding details or whole sections, layering information, cross-linking or extracting portions of articles, and the like only in the electronic version. Authors need to work closely with editors in developing or using such new publication formats and should submit supplementary electronic material for peer review.

Double-spacing all portions of the manuscript— including the title page, abstract, text, acknowledgments, references, individual tables, and legends—and generous margins make it possible for editors and reviewers to edit the text line by line and add comments and queries directly on the paper copy. If manuscripts are submitted electronically, the files should be double-spaced to facilitate printing for reviewing and editing.

Authors should number all of the pages of the manuscript consecutively, beginning with the title page, to facilitate the editorial process.

Reporting Guidelines for Specific Study Designs

Research reports frequently omit important information. Reporting guidelines (www. nlm.nih.gov/services/research_report_guide.html) have been developed for a number of study designs that some journals may ask authors to follow. Authors should consult the Information for Authors of the journal they have chosen.

The general requirements listed in the next section relate to reporting essential elements for all study designs. Authors are encouraged also to consult reporting guidelines relevant to their specific research design. A good source of reporting guidelines is the EQUATOR Network (www.equator-network.org). Specific information about randomized trials can be found at the CONSORT Web site (www.consort-statement.org).

Title Page

The title page should have the following information:

1. *Article title.* Concise titles are easier to read than long, convoluted ones. Titles that are too short may, however, lack important information, such as study design (which is particularly important in identifying randomized, controlled trials). Authors should include all information in the title that will make electronic retrieval of the article both sensitive and specific.

2. *Authors' names and institutional affiliations.* Some journals publish each author's highest academic degree(s), while others do not.

3. The name of the department(s) and institution(s) to which the work should be attributed.

4. Disclaimers, if any.

5. *Contact information for corresponding authors.* The name, mailing address, telephone and fax numbers, and e-mail address of the author responsible for correspondence about the manuscript (the "corresponding author"; this author may or may not be the "guarantor" for the integrity of the study). The corresponding author should indicate clearly whether his or her e-mail address can be published.

6. The name and address of the author to whom requests for reprints should be addressed or a statement that reprints are not available from the authors.

7. Source(s) of support in the form of grants, equipment, drugs, or all of these.

8. *A running head.* Some journals request a short running head or footline, usually no more than 40 characters (including letters and spaces) at the foot of the title page. Running heads are published in most journals but are also sometimes used within the editorial office for filing and locating manuscripts.

9. *Word counts.* A word count for the text only (excluding abstract, acknowledgments, figure legends, and references) allows editors and reviewers to assess whether the information contained in the paper warrants the amount of space devoted to it and whether the submitted manuscript fits within the journal's word limits. A separate word count for the abstract is useful for the same reason.

10. *The number of figures and tables.* It is difficult for editorial staff and reviewers to determine whether the figures and tables that should have accompanied a manuscript were actually included unless the numbers of figures and tables are noted on the title page.

Conflict of Interest Notification Page

To prevent potential conflicts of interest from being overlooked or misplaced, this information needs to be part of the manuscript. The ICMJE has developed a uniform disclosure form for use by ICMJE member journals (www.icmje.org/coi_disclosure. pdf). Other journals are welcome to adopt this form. Individual journals may differ in where they include this information, and some journals do not send information on conflicts of interest to reviewers.

Abstract

Structured abstracts are preferred for original research and systematic reviews. The abstract should provide the context or background for the study and should state the study's purpose, basic procedures (selection of study subjects or laboratory animals, observational and analytical methods), main findings (giving specific effect sizes and their statistical significance, if possible), principal conclusions, and funding sources. It should emphasize the new and important aspects of the study or observations. Articles on clinical trials should contain abstracts that include the items that the CONSORT group has identified as essential (www.consort-statement.org).

Because abstracts are the only substantive portion of the article indexed in many electronic databases, and the only portion many scholars read, authors need to be careful that they accurately reflect the content of the article. Unfortunately, the information contained in many abstracts differs from that in the text. The format required for structured abstracts differs from journal to journal, and some journals use more than one format; authors need to prepare their abstracts in the format specified by the journal they have chosen.

The ICMJE recommends that journals publish the trial registration number at the end of the abstract. It also recommends that, whenever a registration number is available, authors list that number the first time they use a trial acronym to refer to either the trial they are reporting or other trials that they mention in the manuscript.

Introduction

Provide a context or background for the study (i.e., the nature of the problem and its significance). State the specific purpose or research objective of, or hypothesis tested by, the study or observation; the research objective is often more sharply focused when stated as a question. Both the main and secondary objectives should be clear, and any prespecified subgroup analyses should be described. Provide only directly pertinent references, and do not include data or conclusions from the work being reported.

Methods

The Methods section should include only information that was available at the time the plan or protocol for the study was being written; all information obtained during the study belongs in the Results section.

Selection and Description of Participants

Describe your selection of the observational or experimental participants (patients or laboratory animals, including controls) clearly, including eligibility and exclusion criteria and a description of the source population. Because the relevance of such variables as age and sex to the object of research is not always clear, authors should explain their use when they are included in a study report—for example, authors should explain why only participants of certain ages were included or why women were excluded. The guiding principle should be clarity about how and why a study was done in a particular way. When authors use such variables as race or ethnicity, they should define how they measured these variables and justify their relevance.

Technical Information

Identify the methods, apparatus (give the manufacturer's name and address in parentheses), and procedures in sufficient detail to allow others to reproduce the results. Give references to established methods, including statistical methods (see below); provide references and brief descriptions for methods that have been published but are not well-known; describe new or substantially modified methods, give the reasons for using them, and evaluate their limitations. Identify precisely all drugs and chemicals used, including generic name(s), dose(s), and route(s) of administration.

Authors submitting review manuscripts should include a section describing the methods used for locating, selecting, extracting, and synthesizing data. These methods should also be summarized in the abstract.

Statistics

Describe statistical methods with enough detail to enable a knowledgeable reader with access to the original data to verify the reported results. When possible, quantify findings and present them with appropriate indicators of measurement error or uncertainty (such as confidence intervals). Avoid relying solely on statistical hypothesis testing, such as P values, which fail to convey important information about effect size. References for the design of the study and statistical methods should be to standard works when possible (with pages stated). Define statistical terms, abbreviations, and most symbols. Specify the computer software used.

Results

Present your results in logical sequence in the text, tables, and illustrations, giving the main or most important findings first. Do not repeat all the data in the tables or illustrations in the text; emphasize or summarize only the most important observations. Extra or supplementary materials and technical detail can be placed in an appendix where they will be accessible but will not interrupt the flow of the text, or they can be published solely in the electronic version of the journal.

When data are summarized in the Results section, give numeric results not only as derivatives (e.g., percentages) but also as the absolute numbers from which the derivatives were calculated, and specify the statistical methods used to analyze them. Restrict tables and figures to those needed to explain the argument of the paper and to assess supporting data. Use graphs as an alternative to tables with many entries;

do not duplicate data in graphs and tables. Avoid nontechnical uses of technical terms in statistics, such as "random" (which implies a randomizing device), "normal," "significant," "correlations," and "sample."

Where scientifically appropriate, analyses of the data by such variables as age and sex should be included.

Discussion

Emphasize the new and important aspects of the study and the conclusions that follow from them in the context of the totality of the best available evidence. Do not repeat in detail data or other information given in the Introduction or the Results section. For experimental studies, it is useful to begin the discussion by briefly summarizing the main findings, then explore possible mechanisms or explanations for these findings, compare and contrast the results with other relevant studies, state the limitations of the study, and explore the implications of the findings for future research and for clinical practice.

Link the conclusions with the goals of the study but avoid unqualified statements and conclusions not adequately supported by the data. In particular, avoid making statements on economic benefits and costs unless the manuscript includes the appropriate economic data and analyses. Avoid claiming priority or alluding to work that has not been completed. State new hypotheses when warranted, but label them clearly as such.

References

General Considerations Related to References

Although references to review articles can be an efficient way to guide readers to a body of literature, review articles do not always reflect original work accurately. Readers should therefore be provided with direct references to original research sources whenever possible. On the other hand, extensive lists of references to original work on a topic can use excessive space on the printed page. Small numbers of references to key original papers often serve as well as more exhaustive lists, particularly because references can now be added to the electronic version of published papers and because electronic literature searching allows readers to retrieve published literature efficiently.

Avoid using abstracts as references. References to papers accepted but not yet published should be designated as "in press" or "forthcoming"; authors should obtain written permission to cite such papers as well as verification that they have been accepted for publication. Information from manuscripts submitted but not accepted should be cited in the text as "unpublished observations" with written permission from the source.

Avoid citing a "personal communication" unless it provides essential information not available from a public source, in which case the name of the person and date of communication should be cited in parentheses in the text. For scientific articles, obtain written permission and confirmation of accuracy from the source of a personal communication.

Some but not all journals check the accuracy of all reference citations; thus, citation errors sometimes appear in the published version of articles. To minimize such errors, references should be verified using either an electronic bibliographic source, such as PubMed or print copies from original sources. Authors are responsible for checking that none of the references cites retracted articles except in the context of referring to the retraction. For articles published in journals indexed in MEDLINE, the ICMJE considers PubMed (www.pubmed.gov) the authoritative source for information about retractions. Authors can identify retracted articles in MEDLINE using the following search term, where pt in square brackets stands for publication type: Retracted publication [pt] in PubMed.

Reference Style and Format

The Uniform Requirements style for references is based largely on an American National Standards Institute style adapted by the National Library of Medicine (NLM) for its databases. Authors should consult the NLM's *Citing Medicine* (www.ncbi.nlm.nih.gov/books/NBK7256/) for information on its recommended formats for various reference types. Authors may also consult sample references (www.nlm.nih.gov/bsd/uniform_requirements.html), a list of examples extracted from or based on *Citing Medicine* for easy use by the ICMJE audience; these sample references are maintained by the NLM.

References should be numbered consecutively in the order in which they are first mentioned in the text. Identify references in text, tables, and legends by Arabic numerals in parentheses. References cited only in tables or figure legends should be numbered in accordance with the sequence established by the first identification in the text of the particular table or figure. The titles of journals should be abbreviated according to the style used in the list of journals indexed for MEDLINE, posted by the NLM on its Web site (www.nlm.nih.gov/tsd/serials/lji.html). Journals vary on whether they ask authors to cite electronic references within parentheses in the text or in numbered references following the text. Authors should consult with the journal to which they plan to submit their work.

Tables

Tables capture information concisely and display it efficiently; they also provide information at any desired level of detail and precision. Including data in tables rather than text frequently makes it possible to reduce the length of the text.

Type or print each table with double-spacing on a separate sheet of paper. Number tables consecutively in the order of their first citation in the text and supply a brief title for each. Do not use internal horizontal or vertical lines. Give each column a short or an abbreviated heading. Authors should place explanatory matter in footnotes, not in the heading. Explain all nonstandard abbreviations in footnotes, and use the following symbols, in sequence:

*, †, ‡, §, ||, ¶, **, ††, ‡‡, §§, || ||, ¶¶, and so on.

Identify statistical measures of variations, such as standard deviation and standard error of the mean.

Be sure that each table is cited in the text.

If you use data from another published or unpublished source, obtain permission and acknowledge that source fully.

Additional tables containing backup data too extensive to publish in print may be appropriate for publication in the electronic version of the journal, deposited with an archival service, or made available to readers directly by the authors. An appropriate statement should be added to the text to inform readers that this additional information is available and where it is located. Submit such tables for consideration with the paper so that they will be available to the peer reviewers.

Illustrations (Figures)

Figures should be either professionally drawn and photographed, or submitted as photographic-quality digital prints. In addition to requiring a version of the figures suitable for printing, some journals now ask authors for electronic files of figures in a format (e.g., JPEG or GIF) that will produce high-quality images in the Web version of the journal; authors should review the images of such files on a computer screen before submitting them to be sure that meet their quality standards.

For X-ray films, scans, and other diagnostic images as well as pictures of pathology specimens or photomicrographs, send sharp, glossy, black-and-white or color photographic prints, usually 127 mm × 173 mm (5 in × 7 in). Although some journals redraw figures, many do not. Letters, numbers, and symbols on figures should therefore be clear and consistent throughout, and large enough to remain legible when the figure is reduced for publication. Figures should be made as self-explanatory as possible because many will be used directly in slide presentations. Titles and detailed explanations belong in the legends—not on the illustrations themselves.

Photomicrographs should have internal scale markers. Symbols, arrows, or letters used in photomicrographs should contrast with the background.

Photographs of potentially identifiable people must be accompanied by written permission to use the photograph.

Figures should be numbered consecutively in the order they have been cited in the text. If a figure has been published previously, acknowledge the original source and submit written permission from the copyright holder to reproduce the figure. Permission is required irrespective of authorship or publisher except for documents in the public domain.

For illustrations in color, ascertain whether the journal requires color negatives, positive transparencies, or color prints. Accompanying drawings marked to indicate the region to be reproduced might be useful to the editor. Some journals publish illustrations in color only if the author pays the additional cost.

Authors should consult the journal about requirements for figures submitted in electronic formats.

Legends for Illustrations (Figures)

Type or print out legends for illustrations using double-spacing, starting on a separate page, with Arabic numerals corresponding to the illustrations. When symbols, arrows, numbers, or letters are used to identify parts of the illustrations, identify and explain each one clearly in the legend. Explain the internal scale and identify the method of staining in photomicrographs.

Units of Measurement

Measurements of length, height, weight, and volume should be reported in metric units (meter, kilogram, or liter) or their decimal multiples.

Temperatures should be in degrees Celsius. Blood pressures should be in millimeters of mercury, unless other units are specifically required by the journal.

Journals vary in the units they use for reporting hematologic, clinical chemistry, and other measurements. Authors must consult the Information for Authors of the particular journal and should report laboratory information in both local and International System of Units (SI). Editors may request that authors add alternative or non-SI units, as SI units are not universally used. Drug concentrations may be reported in either SI or mass units, but the alternative should be provided in parentheses where appropriate.

Abbreviations and Symbols

Use only standard abbreviations; use of nonstandard abbreviations can be confusing to readers. Avoid abbreviations in the title of the manuscript. The spelled-out abbreviation followed by the abbreviation in parenthesis should be used on first mention unless the abbreviation is a standard unit of measurement.

MANUSCRIPT SUBMISSION

An increasing number of journals now accept electronic submission of manuscripts, whether on disk, as an e-mail attachment, or by downloading directly onto the journal's Web site. Electronic submission saves time and money and allows the manuscript to be handled in electronic form throughout the editorial process (e.g., when it is sent out for review). For specific instructions on electronic submission, authors should consult the journal's Instructions for Authors.

If a paper version of the manuscript is submitted, send the required number of copies of the manuscript and figures; they are all needed for peer review and editing, and the editorial office staff cannot be expected to make the required copies.

Manuscripts must be accompanied by a cover letter, which should include the following information.

- A full statement to the editor about all submissions and previous reports that might be regarded as redundant publication of the same or very similar work. Any such work should be referred to specifically and referenced in the new paper. Copies of such material should be included with the submitted paper to help the editor address the situation.

- A statement of financial or other relationships that might lead to a conflict of interest, if that information is not included in the manuscript itself or in an authors' form.

- A statement that the manuscript has been read and approved by all the authors, the requirements for authorship as stated earlier in this document have been met, and each author believes that the manuscript represents honest work if that information is not provided in another form (see below).

- The name, address, and telephone number of the corresponding author, who is responsible for communicating with the other authors about revisions and final approval of the proofs, if that information is not included in the manuscript itself.

The letter should give any additional information that may be helpful to the editor, such as the type or format of article in the particular journal that the manuscript represents. If the manuscript has been submitted previously to another journal, it is helpful to include the previous editor's and reviewers' comments with the submitted manuscript, along with the authors' responses to those comments. Editors encourage authors to submit these previous communications. Doing so may expedite the review process.

Many journals now provide a presubmission checklist to help the author ensure that all the components of the submission have been included. Some journals now also require that authors complete checklists for reports of certain study types (e.g., the CONSORT checklist at www.consort-statement.org for reports of randomized, controlled trials). Authors should look to see if the journal uses such checklists and send them with the manuscript if they are requested.

Letters of permission to reproduce previously published material, use previously published illustrations, report information about identifiable persons, or to acknowledge people for their contributions must accompany the manuscript.

B   A List of Resources

ADDITIONAL SUGGESTIONS ABOUT STYLE AND PRESENTATION

American Medical Association Manual of Style: A Guide for Authors and Editors. 10th ed. New York, NY: Oxford University Press; 2009.
   The place to go to check on details about punctuation, references, nomenclature, and so on.

Briscoe MH. *Preparing Scientific Illustrations. A Guide to Better Posters, Presentations and Publications.* New York, NY: Springer-Verlag; 1996.
   The title is accurate: The book is full of clear biomedical examples. It is dated, however, so do not look for the latest software tips.

Ross-Larson B. *Edit Yourself. A Manual for Everyone Who Works with Words.* New York, NY: WW Norton & Company; 1996.
   Includes an alphabetized list of commonly misused phrases, such as "It is worth noting that…," that can be eliminated, and others, such as "Draw a comparison between," that should be shortened (to "compare"). Very useful for non–English-speaking writers.

Rothman KJ. Writing for epidemiology. *Epidemiology.* 1998;9:333–337.
   A succinct guide to writing. Although the author emphasizes submissions of epidemiological articles to an epidemiology journal (Epidemiology), his points apply to all of clinical research. If you do not have the patience to read this entire book, at least read this 5-page article.

Taylor RB. *Medical Writing: A Guide for Clinicians, Educators and Researchers,* 2nd ed. New York, NY: Springer; 2011.
   Good ideas from a well-published family physician.

Tufte ER. *The Visual Display of Quantitative Information.* 2nd ed. Cheshire, CT: Graphics Press; 2001.
   Almost a coffee table book. Emphasizes clarity and simplicity. Worth looking at for new ideas.

Wainer H. How to display data badly. *Am Stat.* 1984;38:137–147.
   This article may be hard to find, but it is worth the effort. The author provides 12 rules for making bad figures, including "Change Scales in Mid-Axis" and "More is Murkier: (a) More Decimal Places and (b) More Dimensions."

Young DS, Huth EJ. *SI Units for Clinical Measurement.* Philadelphia, PA: American College of Physicians; 1998.

This is the place to look if you need to convert traditional units into SI (Systeme Internationale) units, or vice versa. It is also a useful source of normal ranges.

Zeiger M. *Essentials of Writing Biomedical Research Papers.* 2nd ed. New York, NY: McGraw-Hill; 1999.

Excellent examples (usually from biomedical, rather than clinical, research) of common mistakes in manuscripts and how to fix them.

SOME SUGGESTED BOOKS ABOUT BIOSTATISTICS

Chernick MR, Friis RH. *Introductory Biostatistics for the Health Sciences: Modern Applications Including Bootstrap.* Hoboken, NJ: John Wiley & Sons; 2003.
Thorough and accessible.

Dawson B, Trapp RG. *Basic & Clinical Biostatistics.* 4th ed. New York, NY: McGraw-Hill; 2004.
This text requires no knowledge of statistics to be useful yet is also remarkably thorough.

van Belle G, Heagerly PJ, Fisher LD, Lumley TS. *Biostatistics. A Methodology for the Health Sciences.* 2nd ed. John Wiley & Sons; 2004.
A complete text covering nearly all the statistical tests most clinical researchers will ever use. Not a casual read.

Glantz SA. *Primer of Biostatistics.* 7th ed. New York, NY: McGraw-Hill; 2012.
A reader-friendly introductory text.

Hosmer DQ, Lemeshow S. *Applied Logistic Regression.* New York, NY: Wiley-Interscience; 2000.
Thorough; more technically advanced than most texts on clinical research.

Jewell NP. *Statistics for Epidemiology.* New York, NY: Chapman & Hall; 2003.
Much of what is discussed also applies to clinical research.

Katz MH. *Multivariable Analysis. A Practical Guide for Clinicians and Public Health Researchers.* 3rd ed. New York, NY: Cambridge University Press; 2011.
The title is accurate: The text is accessible and practical.

Lang TA, Secic M. *How to Report Statistics in Medicine: Annotated Guidelines for Authors, Editors, and Reviewers.* 2nd ed. Philadelphia, PA: American College of Physicians; 2006.
A practical guide that includes chapters on the commonest descriptive and analytic statistics.

Norman GR, Streiner DL. *Biostatistics: The Bare Essentials.* 3rd ed. Hamilton, Ontario: B.C. Decker; 2008.
Well-written, sometimes even humorous, with plenty of examples.

Selvin S. *Statistical Analysis of Epidemiologic Data.* 3rd ed. New York, NY: Oxford University Press; 2004.
Complements more traditional biostatistics texts (e.g., Zar) nicely, with an emphasis on multivariable techniques for dichotomous outcomes.

Vittinghoff E, Glidden DV, Shiboski SC, McCulloch CE. *Regression Methods in Biostatistics: Linear, Logistic, Survival, and Repeated Measures Models.* 2nd ed. New York, NY: Springer-Verlag; 2010.
   A more advanced text that covers regression models.

Zar JH. *Biostatistical Analysis.* 5th ed. New York, NY: Prentice Hall; 2009.
   More oriented to biology than to medicine and clinical research. Requires some statistical knowledge to use; contains lots of formulas and examples.

Index